# — Primary Care —

## A workbook for health professionals

**Alan Gillies**

Radcliffe Medical Press

**Radcliffe Medical Press Ltd**
18 Marcham Road
Abingdon
Oxon OX14 1AA
United Kingdom

**www.radcliffe-oxford.com**
The Radcliffe Medical Press electronic catalogue and online ordering facility.
Direct sales to anywhere in the world.

---

British Library Cataloguing in Publication Data

A catalogue record for this book is available from the British Library.

ISBN 1 85775 936 2

Typeset by Joshua Associates Ltd, Oxford
Printed and bound by TJ International Ltd, Padstow, Cornwall

# Contents

# About this book

Many primary care clinicians are increasingly being faced with the need to incorporate research into their everyday practice. This will vary from being able to read a paper effectively to commissioning their own research. Many will find the language and culture of research offputting.

If you think that research is necessarily esoteric, difficult and remote from primary care, then try this book as an antidote. It is designed as a workbook. It covers 20 topics at the heart of the research agenda in today's NHS. Each topic has its own chapter. They appear to vary in length, but this reflects the on-line resources called in to each topic.

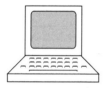

**On-line resource**
This book is actually half of a package. The other half is the Internet site. You will not enjoy reading this book unless you can access the accompanying website:

**http://www.usingresearchinprimarycare.co.uk**

In 1999, when I wrote *Information and IT for Primary Care*, Internet access amongst the NHS was much less common than it is today. The Internet site for that book was an optional extra. For this book, it is an integral part of the whole.

Each time the book calls on an on-line resource you will see the computer symbol.

If you experience problems with an on-line resource link, then check the site for up-to-date information. If there isn't any, please contact the author.

This book is only possible because of the Internet, which has a bad name because of the quality of some of the information found there. However, this book makes use of a large number of resources available and will help you find some really useful information.

All chapters include questions to think about:

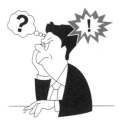

**Questions to think about**

These provide a chance for reflection and reinforce key learning points in each chapter.

Many chapters have practical activities associated with them:

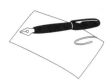

**Practical activities**

Many chapters ask you to evaluate a research study, often on a topic related to the theme of that chapter. Other activities are designed to encourage you to take what you have learned from the book and apply it in your workplace.

**Key points**

At the end of each chapter there are two or three key learning points to reinforce the most important issues for the reader to take away from that chapter.

This is a book about doing: I hope that in the doing, you will both enjoy the experience and learn how to improve your practice.

Alan Gillies
*February 2002*
professor@alangillies.co.uk

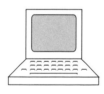

# 1

# Introduction:
# What is good research?

In this introduction, we shall first try to answer the question, 'What is good research?'

**On-line resource**
Visit the website. Find the on-line resources by chapter section. In the Introduction section, you will find a presentation that I gave on R&D to a forum of NHS staff.

View the presentation.

## What criteria can we use to judge good research?

In the workshop presentation, the following criteria were set for designing good research:

- systematic
- reproducible
- designed to eliminate confounding factors
- as simple as possible
- ethical.

When it came to evaluation the following criteria were identified:

- Was there a clearly formulated hypothesis?
- Was a quantitative approach appropriate?
- Is the sample size appropriate?

- What were the biases and have they been minimised?
- Methods – are they appropriate and described in enough detail?
- Methods – what quality control measures were used?
- Are the results credible and significant?
- Conclusions – are they justified?
- Is the research generalisable?

We will explore most of these issues in this book, using a problem-based approach which is currently fashionable within medical curricula.

Many of the following chapters have a journal article associated with them for you to evaluate. In order to facilitate this process we shall first prepare an evaluation framework drawing further upon the research workshop.

In the workshop, I identify four perspectives on research, all found in the NHS:

- the academic perspective
- the practitioner perspective
- the management perspective
- the strategic perspective.

We shall use this as a basis for our evaluation framework. The perspectives were summarised as follows:

| The academic perspective | <ul><li>Research is a *systematic* and *rigorous* process of enquiry</li><li>It seeks to *explain* and *describe*</li><li>It seeks to generate new knowledge and evidence</li><li>It is distinctive from, and complementary to, audit and development</li></ul> |
|---|---|
| The practitioner perspective | <ul><li>Research is about improving the *quality of patient care*</li><li>Research is about *professional development*</li><li>Research is about providing evidence-based care</li></ul> |
| The management perspective | <ul><li>Research is a *requirement* within the modern NHS</li><li>Research funding is drawn from the *patient* budget</li><li>*Spending* on primary and community R&D is set to *double* over the next few years</li><li>NHS R&D has traditionally been concentrated in *secondary* care</li></ul> |
| The strategic perspective | <ul><li>Research is there to investigate the underlying reasons for events</li><li>It has a key role to play within a continuous improvement process</li><li>It sits alongside audit and development activity</li></ul> |

Although traditional research methods courses have emphasised the academic perspective, we shall consider the other perspectives, not least because they are crucial to obtaining funding within the NHS.

At this stage we shall confine our evaluation to relatively high level questions. As we go through the module we will add more detail and techniques which will help you answer the questions in more detail.

## An evaluation checklist for evaluating research articles

Using the above perspectives we can identify the following questions to evaluate a research study.

| | |
|---|---|
| The academic perspective | • Was there a clearly formulated hypothesis?<br>• Was a quantitative approach appropriate?<br>• Is the sample size appropriate?<br>• What were the biases and have they been minimised?<br>• Do the researchers acknowledge the limits of the study?<br>• Methods – are they appropriate and described in enough detail?<br>• Methods – what quality control measures were used?<br>• Are the results credible and significant?<br>• Conclusions – are they justified?<br>• Is the research generalisable? |
| The practitioner perspective | • Is there any obvious application that could lead to an improvement in patient care?<br>• Does the research have relevance to everyday patient care? |
| The management perspective | • Does the research generate evidence that could be disseminated?<br>• Does the article suggest how any resulting evidence could be disseminated?<br>• Would the application of the research have a positive or negative economic impact? |
| The strategic perspective | • Does the research explain the underlying reasons for events?<br>• Will the research assist in the delivery of national NHS strategies? |

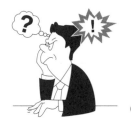

### Questions to think about

1  Do you think there are other perspectives that should be considered?
2  What are the implications of clinical governance for the R&D agenda?
3  Should NHS money be spent on fundamental research with no direct patient benefit?

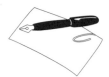

### Practical activities

Use the framework identified above to evaluate the following paper:

• Lattimer V *et al.* (1998) Safety and effectiveness of nurse telephone consultation in out of hours primary care: randomised controlled trial. *BMJ.* **317**: 1054–9.

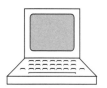

### On-line resource
You can access this paper via the Introduction section of the website. Alternatively, you may like to go straight to:

http://www.bmj.com

You will find Acrobat and Word 97 versions of the evaluation grid on the website.

### Key points

By the end of this chapter, you should be able to:

1  Apply the framework of criteria to a research article.
2  Consider the quality of research from a range of perspectives.

# Part One
# Getting started

# 2

# What is science?

## Introduction

Science is such an all pervasive idea, that we often don't question what science is. 'Good' research is often described as 'scientific'. This chapter attempts to help you understand what 'science' is. In doing so, we shall dabble in dangerous subjects such as philosophy. The section aims to encourage you to examine your own views of what science is, explore some alternatives and then apply these views to health research.

## What is science?

Most people's perceptions of science date from school laboratories and are suitably vague involving experiments and observations. The following is adapted from a piece from the University of Rochester, USA.

### The scientific method

The scientific method is the process by which scientists, collectively and over time, endeavor to construct an accurate (i.e. reliable, consistent and non-arbitrary) representation of the world.

Recognising that personal and cultural beliefs influence both our perceptions and our interpretations of natural phenomena, we aim, through the use of standard procedures and criteria, to minimise those influences when developing a theory. As a famous scientist once said, 'Smart people (like smart lawyers) can come up with very good explanations for mistaken points of view'. In summary, the scientific method attempts to minimise the influence of bias or prejudice in the experimenter when testing an hypothesis or a theory.

The scientific method has four steps:

- observation
- hypothesis formulation
- predictions based upon the hypothesis
- experimental verification or otherwise.

In practice, these may be represented as a cycle (*see* Figure 2.1).

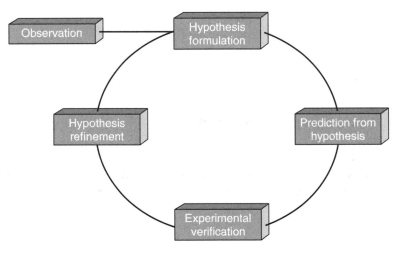

**Figure 2.1**

Once an experiment has been carried out, it is likely that the hypothesis can be refined, which in turn leads to further prediction verification and refinement.

If the experiments bear out the hypothesis it may come to be regarded as a theory or even be described as a law. However, in science it is often said that theories can never be proved, only disproved. There is always the possibility that a new observation or a new experiment will conflict with a long-standing theory.

Experiments may either confirm the hypothesis or refute it. It is an essential part of the scientific method that is testable within a scientific experiment. In physics (and as Lord Kelvin once said, 'physics is science, all else is stamp collecting') as in every experimental science, 'experiment is supreme' and experimental verification of hypothetical predictions is absolutely necessary. Theories which cannot be tested because, for instance, they have no observable ramifications (e.g. a particle whose characteristics make it unobservable) do not qualify as scientific theories. In a truly scientific experiment, only one variable is changed at once and the effect observed.

However, there are many areas of healthcare research where our theories are not testable in a 'scientific' way. Medicine is not generally a science since it deals with people who are complex organisms that do not lend themselves to truly scientific experiments and therefore we must find other ways to remove unwanted effects and minimise bias.

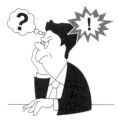

**Questions to think about**

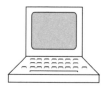

**On-line resource**
Read the 'Ten myths about science' article which can be found in the Chapter 1 section of the website.

1   What has this told you about science?
2   Do you want to disagree?

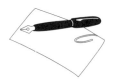

**Practical activities**

Use the framework identified in the Introduction to evaluate the following paper:

- Del Mar CB and Green AC (1995) Aid to diagnosis of melanoma in primary medical care. *BMJ.* **310**: 492–5.

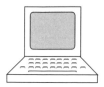

**On-line resource**
You can access this paper via the Introduction section of the website. Alternatively, you may like to go straight to:

http://www.bmj.com

You will find Acrobat and Word 97 versions of the evaluation grid on the website.

**Key points**

By the end of this chapter, you should be able to:

1 Explain what science is and what it isn't.
2 Consider whether a piece of research may be considered 'scientific'.
3 Explain why 'good' research is not necessarily the same as 'scientific' research.

# 3

# The research development lifecycle

## Introduction

The purpose of research within the NHS R&D agenda is to generate new knowledge to improve patient care. As such it is part of a wider range of activities including clinical audit and evidence-based practice.

As a precursor to this chapter, re-visit the methods presentation and look in particular at the section on the relationship between audit and research.

## The relationship between clinical audit, research development and evidence-based practice

Clinical audit, research development and evidence-based practice are all inter-linked within the NHS. Fundamentally, all are concerned with the improvement of patient care.

We shall distinguish between these key terms in the following manner:

- *Research* is about generating new knowledge.
- *Audit* is about improving patient care by ensuring that best existing knowledge and practice is employed.
- *Development* is the application of research findings into a workable format.
- *Evidence-based practice* is clinical practice informed by the best knowledge available.

Strategically, the NHS has placed much emphasis upon trying to capture the potential benefits derived from its expenditure on research.

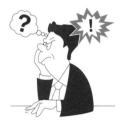

**Questions to think about**

1   How much of your clinical practice is knowingly based upon research evidence?
2   How many times have you changed your practice in recent years in the light of new evidence?

# The research lifecycle

Research is a systematic process. As such we may define a series of stages that we would expect to see in any research study. These may be considered as follows:

- preliminary questions
- defining the research question
- evaluating other work in the field – reviewing the literature
- designing the research study
- analysis of the study
- interpreting the result
- dissemination of the results
- implementation of evidence-based practice.

Much of the rest of the book is concerned with the exploration of these stages. In this chapter we shall consider the preliminary questions.

# Preliminary questions

Before a research study is carried out, it is worth taking stock and considering whether the proposed research study is feasible, economic, significant, generalisable and ethical.

The following questions can be considered as a basic checklist:

---

**Checklist of preliminary questions for any proposed research study**

- Is the problem amenable to research?
- Does it matter?
- Will it provide new knowledge?
- Is it feasible within constraints?
- Can it produce generalisable results?
- Is it ethical?
- Will it be suitable for peer review and publication?

---

If the answer to any of these questions is 'No', then the work is not worth pursuing in its current form, although it may be possible in a different form.

There are other reasons why we might not proceed with a research study. However, these require further work. It should simply be noted that a set of 'Yes' answers at this stage is only an indication that the problem is worthy of further study. For example, it is possible that after consulting the literature, it is found that the work has already been done elsewhere.

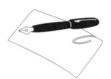

### Practical activities

Use the framework identified in the Introduction to evaluate the following paper:

- Smith T, Moore EHJ and Tunstall-Pedoe H (1997) Review by a local medical research ethics committee of the conduct of approved research projects, by examination of patients' case notes, consent forms, and research records and by interview. *BMJ*. **314**: 1588.

### On-line resource
You can access this paper via the Chapter 3 section of the website. Alternatively, you may like to go straight to:

http://www.bmj.com

You will find Acrobat and Word 97 versions of the evaluation grid on the website.

**Key points**

By the end of this chapter, you should be able to:

1 Distinguish between audit, research and development.
2 Discuss how effective the emphasis on these activities has been in improving your clinical practice.
3 Evaluate basic questions about a research study to test its feasibility and usefulness.

# 4

# Identifying a research problem

## Introduction

In this chapter we shall consider the problem of the research question. It is worthwhile being mindful of the words of Deep Thought from the late and much lamented Douglas Adams' cult classic *The Hitchhiker's Guide to the Galaxy* (*see* Figure 3.1).

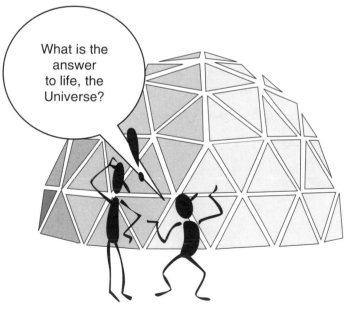

**Figure 3.1**

In *The Hitchhiker's Guide to the Galaxy*, Deep Thought claims the answer is 42. More importantly, he justifies this by claiming that the people posing the questions had never really defined the question correctly.

## Refining the question

As in the fictional case above, the problem with research questions is that they can be rather broad. Research questions need to be precise, tractable and amenable to investigation. This is generally achieved through a process of refinement.

Consider for example the following question, 'Does a computer in a general practice improve patient care?'.

This is a question that may reasonably be asked in the light of the £6 billion investment in information technology (IT) made by the NHS since 1990. However, the question as it stands is far too broad to be investigated. To refine it, we must seek to investigate the following issues:

- What factors may be considered as having an impact on the quality of patient care? These are known as confounding factors.
- How do we measure an improvement in patient care?

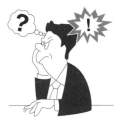 **Questions to think about**

'Does a computer in a general practice improve patient care?'

Complete the following table (the first has been done for you to get you started)

| Confounding factors | Measures of improvements in patient care |
|---|---|
| Number of clinicians in practice | % target population BP measured |
|  |  |
|  |  |
|  |  |
|  |  |
|  |  |

What other ambiguities can you spot in this question?

Another way of helping to refine a research question is to think in terms of aims and objectives. In this approach:

- the *aim* is a single statement that states the purpose of the research succinctly
- the *objectives* describe a series of tasks which, if completed, would enable the aim to be met.

When a PhD student starts, I often ask them to complete the following statement:

'The aim of my PhD project is . . .', in not more than 15 words, much in the manner of a competition tie-breaker.

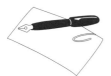

### Practical activities

1 For the studies you have read in this book so far, consider the stated objectives and see how they are met.

- Lattimer V *et al.* (1998) Safety and effectiveness of nurse telephone consultation in out of hours primary care: randomised controlled trial. *BMJ.* **317**: 1054–9.
- Del Mar CB and Green AC (1995) Aid to diagnosis of melanoma in primary medical care. *BMJ.* **310**: 492–5.
- Smith T, Moore EJH and Tunstall-Pedoe H (1997) Review by a local medical research ethics committee of the conduct of approved research projects, by examination of patients' case notes, consent forms, and research records and by interview. *BMJ.* **314**: 1588.

*Note*: The use of the term 'objective' in a *BMJ* structured abstract corresponds to the term 'aim' as used in this chapter.

2 Use the framework identified in the Introduction to evaluate the following paper:

- Spitzer RL, Kroenke K, Williams JBW and the Patient Health Questionnaire Primary Care Study Group (1999) Validation and utility of a self-report version of PRIME-MD the PHQ primary care study. *JAMA.* **282**: 1737–44.

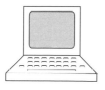

### On-line resource

You can access this paper via the Chapter 4 section of the website.

You will find Acrobat and Word 97 versions of the evaluation grid on the website.

3 Choose a topic for investigation from your work, then:

- frame a general research question within this topic area
- identify confounding factors and how the property under investigation may be measured
- write a more precise research question in terms of a 'The aim of my research is to . . .' statement
- identify a set of objectives to meet this aim.

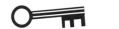 **Key points**

By the end of this section, you should be able to:

1 Identify and refine a research question.
2 Consider confounding factors.
3 Describe the aim of a research study in a short succinct statement.

# 5

# The ethics of research

## Introduction

The ethical issues around health research are many and complex. In this chapter we can merely introduce the main issues. In healthcare research, it is often assumed that the ethics of health research can be reduced to satisfying the local research ethics committee.

## The process of gaining ethical approval

The *NHSE North West Regional R&D Handbook* has the following advice on this process.

### *Overview*

When planning clinical research, you should always pay careful attention to the ethical issues which may result from your work. Clinical research generally involves the participation of patients, staff, healthy volunteers or students, and ethical and legal issues are therefore likely to be raised. To ensure that patients and others are protected, Local Research Ethics Committees (LRECs), usually administered by health authorities, have been put in place, working to nationally published guidelines. LRECs are primarily concerned with the welfare and dignity of the participants of any research project, as well as the validity of the study. The LREC ensures that individuals are not tested unnecessarily and are not misinformed or ill-treated. If your study involves the participation of students, you may require ethical approval from the institute providing your student population, in addition to approval from your LREC.

## Role of the Local Research Ethics Committee

The LRECs are usually organised geographically by health district and their purpose is 'to consider the ethics of proposed research projects which will involve human subjects and which will take place broadly within the NHS'. They are also concerned with the quality and integrity of a project. The guidelines issued by the Department of Health in *Health Service Guideline (91)5* state that any research involving the following requires ethical approval:

- NHS patients (past or present)
- Foetal material and *in vitro* fertilisation involving NHS patients
- The recently dead, in NHS premises
- Access to records of past or present NHS patients
- The use of, or potential access to, NHS premises or facilities.

## Application procedure

The appropriate LREC should be contacted in the initial stages of protocol development if there is any doubt about whether ethical approval is required. Certain types of research (e.g. laboratory-based studies) may be exempt from the need for LREC approval, but you should check on this before starting work. You may find that both your employing organisation and your research sponsor require written ethical approval or a waiver from the requirements of ethical approval. Early contact with the administrator of the LREC is also advised in order to check the dates of meetings and submission dates. In order to gain ethical approval, an application form should be completed; the form can be obtained from the secretary to the ethics committee. Forms may vary between LRECs, but most will have questions which fall into the following categories:

- project title
- names and details of investigators
- study objectives
- outline of study design
- scientific background to study
- recruitment details
- tests, instruments, drugs and devices to be used
- GPs' consent
- potential discomfort and risks to subjects
- informed consent (consent form and patient information sheet)
- indemnity from drug or equipment suppliers
- cost and sponsor payment details.

When applying for ethical approval, it is important to remember that some members of the ethics committee are lay members and there may not be a member who is a specialist in your area of research. Therefore, it is necessary for the document to be non-technical and readable. When assessing the application the LREC will look for the following points:

- any possible effects on the individuals' health
- the scientific merit of the project
- possible hazards and proposed ways of handling them
- expected degree of discomfort or distress for the participants
- adequate supervision from suitably qualified and experienced personnel
- inducements to be offered to patients or the investigators
- suitability of the information sheet
- procedures for obtaining consent from the subjects or, where necessary, their parents or guardians
- measures in place to ensure subject confidentiality.

If you do receive ethical approval, this does not give authorisation for the project to proceed. The project still requires approval from the organisation(s) in which you intend to carry out the research.

## *Points to consider*

### *Recruitment*

Potential subjects should never be coerced or made to take part in a study against their will. The investigators should emphasise the fact that participation is voluntary and that participants can withdraw from the study at any time without detriment to their treatment. It is the responsibility of the researchers to ensure that the participants have no contraindications to the study.

### *Obtaining participant consent*

Written informed consent is required from all participants and the LREC will want evidence that a volunteer will be given enough information to provide this. Both a written and verbal explanation of the study is usually required before the participant signs the consent form. Some LRECs have a standard consent form which should be used in conjunction with the information sheet. Items to include on the patient information sheet are:

- the purpose of the study
- details of the procedures involved and what is required of the participants
- length of the study
- any effect on patients' treatment by participating in the trial

- any potential harmful effects or discomfort they may have as well as any potential benefits
- assurance of confidentiality and compliance with the Data Protection Act.

Tips on designing an information sheet are:

- use short sentences
- avoid jargon and medical terms, or explain such language when used
- wherever possible, use lists or bullet points instead of paragraphs
- use subheadings
- use a minimum of 12-point font size.

Make sure it is easy to read, several versions in different languages may be needed. It may be appropriate to use a question-and-answer format (Wager *et al.*, 1995). Some studies require the use of participants who may find it difficult or impossible to give informed consent, e.g. the elderly or children. In these cases, the LREC will seek the appropriate specialist advice. Multi-Centre Research Ethics Committees (MRECs) have been set up to give approval to studies that are multi-centre, spread over regions, and involve five or more LRECs. If an MREC approves a multi-centre study, the application must still be submitted to the LRECs for all the research sites. The LREC may then approve or reject the study, but on local study groups only. For further details about the MREC, contact the appropriate MREC administrator (their address can be obtained from your LREC office).

## *Research on animals*

A Home Office licence is required for any experiments involving animals. Your Trust may have its own rules and regulations about the conduct of animal work on its premises.

## *Reference*

- Wager E, Tooley PJH, Emanuel MB and Wood S (1995) How to do it: get patients' consent to enter clinical trials. *BMJ.* **31**: 734–7.

Taken from the *NHSE North West Regional R&D Handbook*.
URL: http://www.doh.gov.uk/pub/docs/doh/rdhandbook.pdf

The role of ethics committees is a valid and important one. However, there are a number of problems inherent in the system:

- it tends to reduce ethical considerations to a paper exercise
- it tends to push the responsibility away from the researcher onto the ethics committee.

The responsibility to do ethical research rests with the individual researcher, not with an external body.

## What is ethical research?

Consider the following proposition:

*All control trials are fundamentally unethical as patients are treated unequally. In the case where a treatment is advantageous, the control group is denied a potential benefit. In the case where a treatment is disadvantageous, the active group is exposed to a risk. We cannot obtain truly informed consent from the patients because we do not know in advance the nature of the risk.*

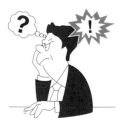

**Questions to think about**

1  What are the ethical principles raised in this argument?
2  Do you agree with the argument made? Justify your answer.
3  On what ethical grounds may randomised controlled trials be justified?
4  How would you feel if you were asked to take part in a randomised controlled trial (RCT)? Would the grounds you have identified in 3 above convince you to take part or not? Why?

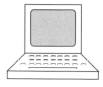

**On-line resource**
For further reading, see the website where you will find a link to the complete *North West Regional R&D Handbook*, and the National Bioethics Advisory Commission's report from the USA.

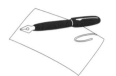

### Practical activities

1 Read the following paper:

- Schultz WW, van Andel P, Sabelis I and Mooyaart E (1999) Magnetic resonance imaging of male and female genitals during coitus and female sexual arousal. *BMJ*. **319**: 1596–1600.

Imagine you are on the local research ethics committee, and you have been asked by your colleagues to review this as a proposal, before the research has been carried out. What are the key ethical issues in the study, based upon the issues highlighted above, that the LREC might consider, as well as any other that you feel are relevant.

2 Use the framework identified in the Introduction to evaluate the following paper:

- Smith T, Moore EJH and Tunstall-Pedoe H (1997) Review by a local medical research ethics committee of the conduct of approved research projects, by examination of patients' case notes, consent forms, and research records and by interview. *BMJ*. **314**: 1588.

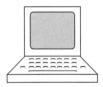

### On-line resource

You can access this paper via the Chapter 5 section of the website. Alternatively, you may like to go straight to:

http://www.bmj.com

You will find Acrobat and Word 97 versions of the evaluation grid on the website.

### Key points

By the end of this chapter, you should be able to:

1 Prepare with assistance an application to a local ethics committee.
2 Discuss the ethical principles underpinning research.

# 6

# Literature review

## Introduction

Before starting this chapter, please read the following articles as examples of literature searches in different media:

- Buetow SA, Sibbald B, Cantrill JA and Halliwell S (1996) Prevalence of potentially inappropriate long term prescribing in general practice in the United Kingdom, 1980–95: systematic literature review. *BMJ*. **313**: 1371–4.
- Kim P, Eng TR, Deering MJ and Maxfield A (1999) Published criteria for evaluating health related websites: review. *BMJ*. **318**: 647–9.
- Sullivan F and Mitchell E (1995) Has general practitioner computing made a difference to patient care? A systematic review of published reports. *BMJ*. **311**: 848–52.
- Greenhalgh T (2000) Papers that summarise other papers (systematic reviews and meta-analyses). In: *How to Read a Paper (2e)*. BMJ Books, London.

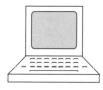

**On-line resource**
You will be able to access these papers via the Chapter 6 section of the website. Alternatively, you may like to go straight to:

http://www.bmj.com

## Literature review

The purpose of the literature review is to investigate the following questions:

- Has the problem already been investigated?
- Has the question been adequately answered already?
- If not, what parts of the question have been satisfactorily answered?

The principal tool for searching the medical literature remains the Medline database provided by the National Library of Medicine in Washington DC. The remainder of this chapter will seek to give you a working knowledge of tools to identify and access the literature.

# Tools available on-line

## *The virtual library*

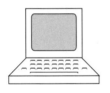

**On-line resource**
You can access the virtual library via the Chapter 6 section of the website. Alternatively, you may like to go straight to:

http://www.healthlibrary.org.uk

or

http://www.healthinformatics.org.uk/Vlibrary/

The virtual library is an on-line library designed by the author to be easy and fun to use:

- it looks like a library
- it is full of books, journals and databases
- it links to other libraries in the world
- it has a cellar for you to burrow around in.

When you enter the library you find yourself in the entrance hall:

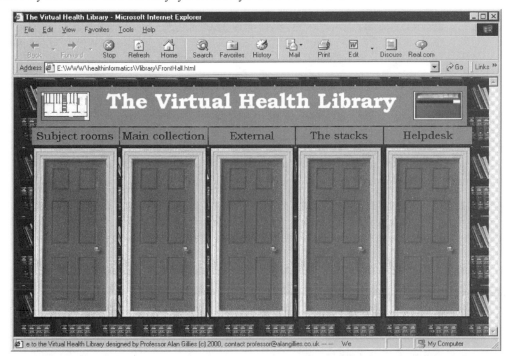

If you move the mouse across a door it will open for you:

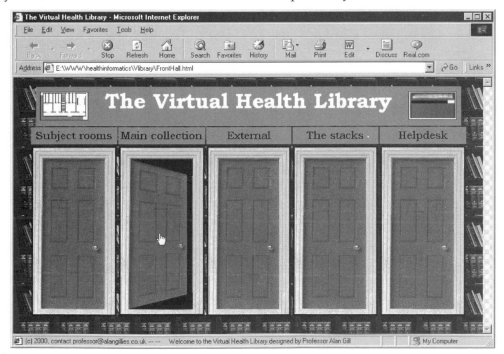

We will only show you the main collection, and leave the rest for you to find.

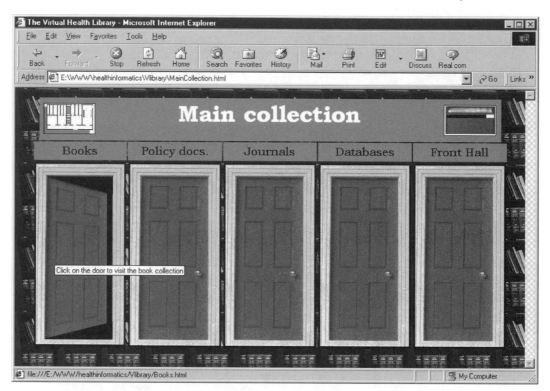

The books section has eight textbooks covering topics such as:

- statistics
- epidemiology
- qualitative methods
- reading research papers
- dermatology.

When you move across a book, it opens. To read it, click on the open book:

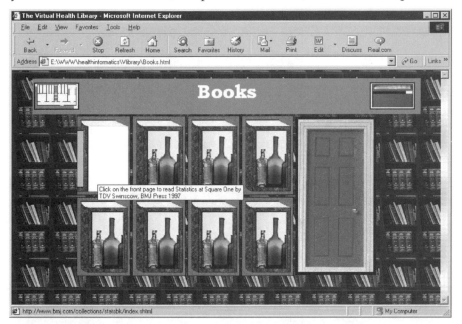

To leave the room, click on the door:

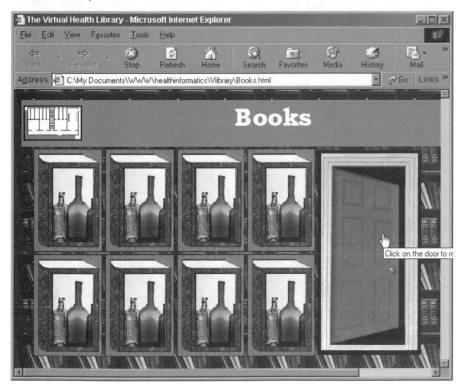

The policy documents section contains many useful policy documents from the UK NHS over the last few years.

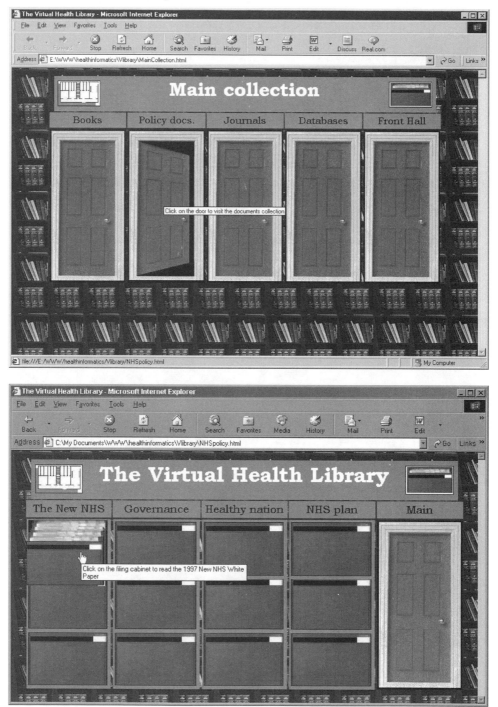

Documents in this section include:

- *The New NHS* White Paper (1997)
- *The NHS Plan* (2000).

However, other sections of the library provide wider access. For example, the informatics room provides access to information strategy documents for England, Wales and Scotland. Via links to the Department of Health, you can obtain almost any recent publication.

The journals section features key journals from medicine and nursing, as well as a list of almost all journals available free on-line:

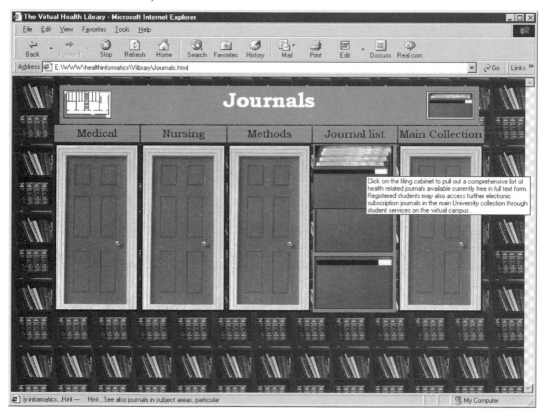

To access the *BMJ*, used extensively in this text, use the medical door and click on the cover:

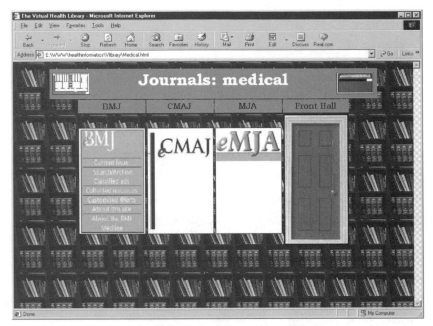

The on-line version of the *BMJ* appears in its own window. I'll let you find this for yourself, as I don't wish to abuse anybody's copyright!

By now you may want to find a quick way around the library. Try clicking on the map at the top left of the screen:

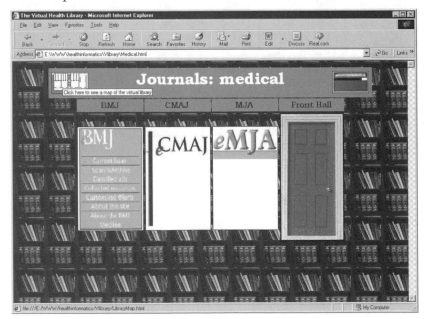

This is a clever map: not only does it tell you where you are, but by clicking on a room you can go there. Eat your heart out Star Trek!

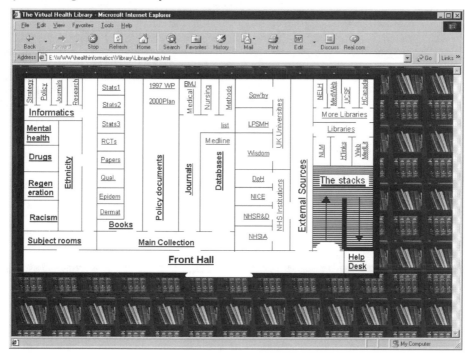

For example, click on the database room and you will go there:

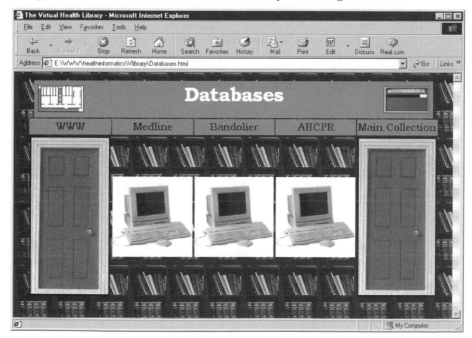

Move across the PCs and they come on:

The Virtual Health Library - Microsoft Internet Explorer

File   Edit   View   Favorites   Tools   Help

Back   Forward   Stop   Refresh   Home   Search   Favorites   Media   History   Mail   Print   Edit

Address  C:\My Documents\WWW\healthinformatics\Vlibrary\Databases.html     Go   Links

# Databases

| WWW | Medline | Bandolier | AHCPR | Main Collection |

For example, the left hand PC gives access to Medline, the database of published articles held in Washington at the National Library of Medicine. Click on this PC to access the Medline database. For now we shall go there, but we shall return to the library in the practical exercises at the end of the chapter.

## Medline

Before you explore the Medline database, first read the following article:

• Greenhalgh T (2000) The Medline database. In: *How to Read a Paper (2e)*. BMJ Books, London.

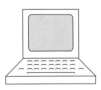

**On-line resource**
You can access this article via the Chapter 6 section of the website. Alternatively, you may like to go straight to:

http://www.bmj.com

or go back to the books section of the virtual library, where you will find the book *How to Read a Paper*.

When you click on the Medline PC, a new window opens on your screen containing the PubMed access to Medline:

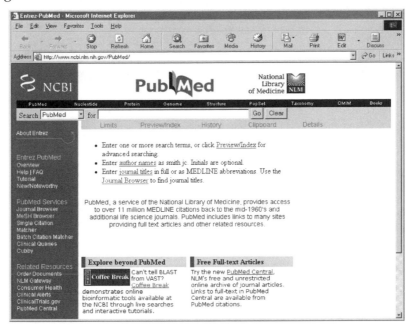

Let us suppose that we wish to find articles relating to diabetes in primary care. We enter the key terms in the search window:

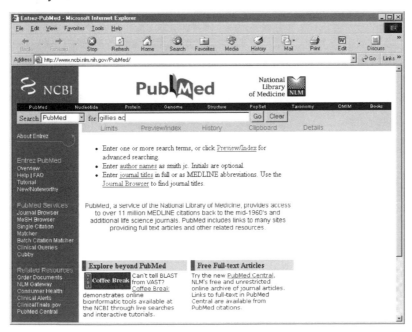

and then click on 'Go'.

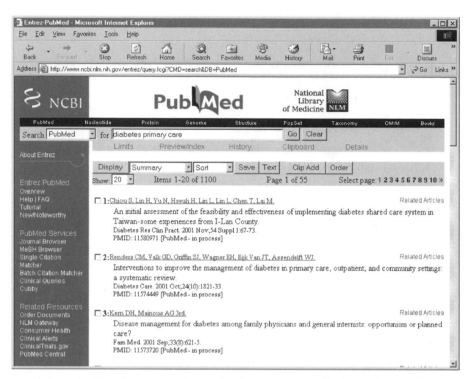

If we are interested in the second article then we can click on the authors' names:

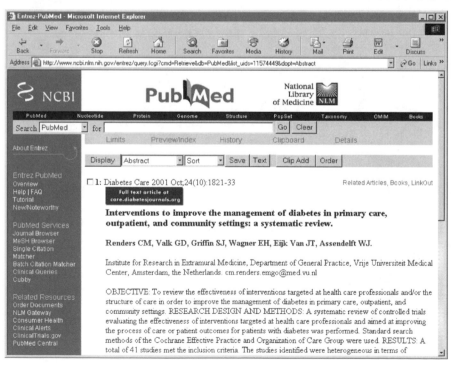

Medline only provides abstracts of articles, but will supply links to full text on-line where available. Be warned, they are not all free! Click on the 'Full text article' box here and you will be asked to pay:

You may prefer to use the citation details to obtain the article elsewhere, for example from a postgraduate medical centre.

---

Renders CM, Valk GD, Griffin SJ *et al.* (2001) Interventions to improve the management of diabetes in primary care, outpatient, and community settings: a systematic review. *Diabetes Care.* **24**(10): 1821–33 (Institute for Research in Extramural Medicine, Department of General Practice, Vrije Universiteit Medical Center, Amsterdam, The Netherlands. cm.renders.emgo@med.vu.nl)

**Objective**: To review the effectiveness of interventions targeted at healthcare professionals and/or the structure of care in order to improve the management of diabetes in primary care, outpatient and community settings.

**Research design and methods**: A systematic review of controlled trials evaluating the effectiveness of interventions targeted at healthcare professionals and aimed at improving the process of care or patient outcomes for patients with diabetes was performed. Standard search methods of the Cochrane Effective Practice and Organisation of Care Group were used.

**Results**: A total of 41 studies met the inclusion criteria. The studies identified were heterogeneous in terms of interventions, participants, settings, and reported outcomes. In all studies, the interventions were multifaceted. The interventions were targeted at healthcare professionals only in 12 studies, at the organisation of care only in nine studies, and at both in 20 studies. Complex professional interventions improved the process of care, but the effect on patient outcomes remained less clear because such outcomes were rarely assessed. Organisational interventions that facilitated the structured and regular review of patients also showed a favourable effect on process measures. Complex interventions in which patient education was added and/or the role of a nurse was enhanced, led to improvements in patient outcomes as well as the process of care.

**Conclusions**: Multifaceted professional interventions and organisational interventions that facilitate structured and regular review of patients were effective in improving the process of care. The addition of patient education to these interventions and the enhancement of the role of nurses in diabetes care, led to improvements in patient outcomes and the process of care.

Now you can practise your skills with the following exercises:

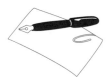

### Practical activities

1 Carry out a literature search to investigate existing literature work investigating whether the introduction of computers has benefited cervical screening using Medline.

   One of the key issues here is the prevalence of papers in the US literature on automatic smear analysis. We are more interested in papers on the use of computers to encourage patients to attend for smear tests.

   To address this problem, the [More like this] feature associated with the following article:

   • Robson J *et al.* (1995) Audit of preventive activities in 16 inner London practices using a validated measure of patient population, the 'active patient' denominator. Healthy Eastenders Project. *Br J Gen Pract.* **45**: 463–6.

   produces the following list (first 20 only!):

- Robson J *et al.* (1995) Audit of preventive activities in 16 inner London practices using a validated measure of patient population, the 'active patient' denominator. Healthy Eastenders Project. *Br J Gen Pract.* **45**: 463–6.
- Scobie S *et al.* (1995) Can general practice data be used for needs assessment and healthcare planning in an inner-London district? *J Public Health Med.* **17**: 475–83.
- Lervy B *et al.* (1994) Practice characteristics associated with audit activity: a medical audit advisory group survey. *Br J Gen Pract.* **44**: 311–14.
- Hearnshaw H *et al.* (1998) A survey of audit activity in general practice. *Br J Gen Pract.* **48**: 979–81.
- Lawrence M *et al.* (1990) A total audit of preventive procedures in 45 practices caring for 430,000 patients. *BMJ.* **300**: 1501–3.
- Mant D *et al.* (1986) Can the prevalence of disease risk factors be assessed from general practice records? *BMJ.* (Clin Res Ed). **292**: 102–4.
- Whitelaw FG *et al.* (1996) Completeness and accuracy of morbidity and repeat prescribing records held on general practice computers in Scotland. *Br J Gen Pract.* **46**: 181–6.
- Wilson AD (1987) Cervical cytology: a general practice audit. *Fam Pract.* **4**: 56–60.
- Weingarten MA *et al.* (1989) Computerized protocol for preventive medicine: a controlled self-audit in family practice. *Fam Pract.* **6**: 120–4.
- Atri J *et al.* (1996) Fair shares in healthcare? Ethnic and socioeconomic influences on recording of preventive care in selected inner London general practices. Healthy Eastenders Project. *BMJ.* **312**: 614–17.
- Phillips A *et al.* (1987) Feasibility of contact surveys in general practice. *BMJ* (Clin Res Ed). **295**: 1101–4.
- Griffiths C *et al.* (1994) Registration health checks: inverse care in the inner city? *Br J Gen Pract.* **44**: 201–4.
- Pringle M *et al.* (1995) Assessment of the completeness and accuracy of computer medical records in four practices committed to recording data on computer. *Br J Gen Pract.* **45**: 537–41.
- Robson J *et al.* (1989) Using nurses for preventive activities with computer assisted follow-up: a randomised controlled trial. *BMJ.* **298**: 433–6.
- Jones B *et al.* (1999) Improving preventive practice. An educational intervention using chart audit. *Aust Fam Physician.* **28** (suppl 1): S41–5.
- Majeed FA *et al.* (1994) Using patient and general practice characteristics to explain variations in cervical smear uptake rates. *BMJ.* **308**: 1272–6.
- Lawrence M *et al.* (1994) Auditing audits: use and development of the Oxfordshire Medical Audit Advisory Group rating system. *BMJ.* **309**: 513–16.
- Harriss C *et al.* (1994) Do general practice computer systems assist in medical audit? *Fam Pract.* **11**: 51–6.

- Brotons C *et al.* (1996) Evaluation of preventive and health promotion activities in 166 primary care practices in Spain. The Coordinating Group For Prevention and Health Promotion in Primary Care in Spain. *Fam Pract.* **13**: 144–51.
- Holden J *et al.* (1996) An audit of 319 deaths across four general practices. *Br J Clin Pract.* **50**: 79–80.

2 Medline produces only abstracts, however, the journal archives in the virtual library, e.g. *BMJ*, produce full text articles. Only one of these articles falls into the group covered by the archive.

Investigate the same topic using the *BMJ* archive, applying two strategies:

- start with the 1994 Majeed paper and look for similar papers, or papers, that have cited this paper
- a general search strategy using keywords to identify target papers.

Compare the results.

For example, this paper has been cited by the following papers:

- Majeed FA, Chaturvedi N, Reading R and Ben-Shlomo Y (1994) Equity in the NHS: monitoring and promoting equity in primary and secondary care. *BMJ*. **308**: 1426–9
- Moser K, Naish J and Chambers M (1994) Cervical smear uptake rates. *BMJ*. **309**: 476–7.
- Majeed FA, Cook DG, Poloniecki J *et al.* (1995) Sociodemographic variables for general practices: use of census data. *BMJ*. **310**: 1373–4.
- Majeed FA, Cook DG, Poloniecki J *et al.* (1995) Using data from the 1991 census. *BMJ*. **310**: 1511–14.
- Scrivener G and Lloyd D (1995) Allocating census data to general practice populations: implications for study of prescribing variation at practice level. *BMJ* **311**: 163–5.
- Majeed FA, Voss S (1995) Performance indicators for general practice. *BMJ* **311**: 209–10.
- Aylin P, Majeed FA and Cook DG (1996) Home visiting by general practitioners in England and Wales. *BMJ*. **313**: 207–10.
- Sturdy P, Nash J, Carter Y and Griffiths C (1996) Study in London confirms influence of ethnic group on treatment for asthma. *BMJ* **313**: 1260.
- Pollock AM, Vickers N (1998) Deprivation and emergency admissions for cancers of colorectum, lung, and breast in South East England: ecological study. *BMJ*. **317**: 245–52.
- Reid FDA, Cook DG and Majeed A (1999) Explaining variation in hospital admission rates between general practices: cross sectional study. *BMJ*. **319**: 98–103.

3 Use the framework identified in the Introduction to evaluate the following paper:

- Egger M, Davey Smith G, Schneider M and Minder C (1997) Bias in meta-analysis detected by a simple, graphical test. *BMJ.* **315**: 629–34.

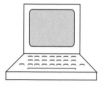

**On-line resource**
You can access this paper via the Chapter 6 section of the website. Alternatively, you may like to go straight to:

http://www.bmj.com

You will find Acrobat and Word 97 versions of the evaluation grid on the website.

4 See if you can find the following in the virtual library:

- *Information for Health*
- Caldicott Report on patient confidentiality
- The Department of Health site
- The National Electronic Library for Health
- WebMedLit.

 **Key points**

By the end of this chapter, you should be able to:

1 Access and navigate the virtual library.
2 Access and interrogate the Medline database.
3 Carry out a literature search on a topic of your choice.

# Part Two
# Methods for
# quantitative research

# 7

# Data analysis, random and control trials

## Introduction

Random control trials are the single most important design method in medicine, and we need to understand how they work. Therefore, before starting this chapter, please read the following sections from *How to Read a Paper* by Trisha Greenhalgh:

- Getting your bearings (deciding what the paper is about)
- Papers that report diagnostic or screening tests
- Papers that report drug trials
- Statistics for the non-statistician
- Statistics for the non-statistician II: 'Significant' relations and their pitfalls
- Assessing the methodological quality of published papers

Also read the following (mainly short) articles by way of introduction to this topic:

- Altman DG and Bland JM (1999) How to randomise. *BMJ*. **319**: 703–4.
- Torgerson DJ and Roberts C (1999) Understanding controlled trials: Randomisation methods: concealment. *BMJ*. **319**: 375–6.
- Roberts C and Torgerson DJ (1999) Understanding controlled trials: Baseline imbalance in randomised controlled trials. *BMJ*. **319**: 185.
- Edwards SJL, Braunholtz DA, Lilford RJ and Stevens AJ (1999) Ethical issues in the design and conduct of cluster randomised controlled trials. *BMJ*. **318**: 1407–9.
- Altman DG and Bland JM (1999) Treatment allocation in controlled trials: why randomise? *BMJ*. **318**: 1209.

- Roberts C and Torgerson DJ (1998) Understanding controlled trials: Randomisation methods in controlled trials. *BMJ*. **317**: 1301–10.
- Campbell MK and Grimshaw JM (1998) Cluster randomised trials: time for improvement. *BMJ*. **317**: 1171–2.
- Kunz R and Oxman AD (1998) The unpredictability paradox: review of empirical comparisons of randomised and non-randomised clinical trials. *BMJ*. **317**: 1185–90.
- Edwards SJL, Lilford RJ and Hewison J (1998) The ethics of randomised controlled trials from the perspectives of patients, the public, and healthcare professionals. *BMJ*. **317**: 1209–12.
- Roberts C and Sibbald B (1998) Understanding controlled trials: Randomising groups of patients. *BMJ*. **316**: 1898–1900.

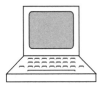

**On-line resource**
You can access these papers via the Chapter 7 section of the website. Alternatively, you may like to go straight to:

http://www.bmj.com

# Understanding a random control trial in detail

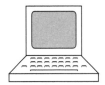

**On-line resource**
Read the following paper which details a random control trial from general practice:

Hamilton W, Round A and Sharp D (1999) Effect on hospital attendance rates of giving patients a copy of their referral letter: randomised controlled trial. *BMJ*. **318**: 1392–5.

In order to tackle the questions below, also refer to:

Altman DG and Bland JM (1999) Statistics notes: how to randomise. *BMJ*. **319**: 703–4.

You can access these papers via the Chapter 7 section of the website. Alternatively, you may like to go straight to:

http://www.bmj.com

Consider the trial profile (*see* Figure 7.1) shown below and then consider the questions to think about.

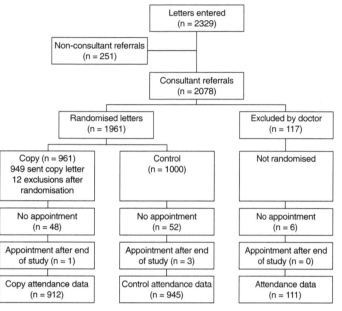

**Figure 7.1**

**Questions to think about**

1   Do you accept the randomisation strategy in this case?
2   Do the exclusions have a significant impact upon the generalisability of this study?
3   Do you agree with the conclusions?
4   Consider the claim: *This is the largest prospective study of non-attendance at outpatient departments.* Is this true? Can you find any other studies of this type in Medline?
5   The authors assert:

*The results do not support the hypothesis that sending patients a copy of their referral letter reduces non-attendance, despite earlier work suggesting that this might be so.*

Look up reference 21 in the *BMJ* archive. What differences can you spot to account for this different conclusion?

6   They also claim:

*The suggestion that non-attendance reflects inadequate communication between doctor and patient supported by the results. The study shows the importance of performing a full randomised controlled trial rather than relying on impressions from underpowered pilot studies.*

Do you agree with this?

7   Consider the following assertion:

*The non-attendance rate of 5.3% is low compared with previous studies, was similar to non-study doctors concurrently. The patients excluded from the randomisation cannot explain this; there were few, and they had a low non-attendance rate, probably reflecting the conditions that led to their exclusion from randomisation.*

Do you agree?

8   Do you agree with the following?

*Nor can the seven mismatches between the attendance record in the doctor notes and the hospital data fully explain the low recorded non-attendance rate. The doctor record was used as the gold standard, in that a consultant's reply letter is unequivocal evidence of attendance, whereas other studies quote hospital data, which will contain these small inaccuracies.*

9   On the possible effects of a copy letter, the authors assert that:

*A referral letter may not contain the information that a patient needs to decide if attendance is worthwhile; conversely, it may inform some patients such that they consider attendance unnecessary. In the case of a referral made primarily for reassurance, the copy letter alone may provide this. Although such reassurance might decrease attendance, this effect should increase cancellations rather than non-attendances. It is possible two effects are operating in different directions: increased attendance (in those whose understanding of their condition and thus the need for an appointment is improved) and increased non-attendance (in those reassured by the letter who decide not to attend). On the other hand, it may simply be that any effect of the copy letter is lost by the time of the appointment, on average ten weeks later. A copy may have to be sent nearer to the time of the appointment to be effective. The copy letter is not without value, however. Theoretically it empowers patients; it was certainly not seen as undesirable by patients, given the lack of adverse comments. This supports the findings of the pilot study, which showed that patients find copy letters helpful. Previous studies have shown the acceptability of sending patients a copy of the consultant's reply to their general practitioner, but none has studied a copy of the general practitioner's letter to the consultant. The low rate of excluded patients and the doctors' replies to the questionnaire show that they also accept the concept. Several saw provision of a copy as a logical extension of patients' access to their records. The discipline of knowing that the patient may receive a copy could have improved the letter's accuracy, as only three patients sought to have inaccuracies corrected. This can be compared with accuracy levels of 63–95% when letters are assessed by doctors, and 43% when assessed by patients.*

Do you agree with this argument?

10 Their overall conclusion is:

*Non-attendance remains an important issue for doctors and their patients. Despite the negative results of this study, the possibility of applying interventions in primary care to reduce non-attendance still exists. Primary care groups will be well placed to advise on which interventions are likely to be best for their populations.*

In the light of this conclusion is the paper helpful to primary care groups (PCGs)?

11 Do you agree with the authors' three key messages:

- copy letters to the patient do not decrease non-attendance at hospital outpatients
- the concept of copying letters to patients is acceptable to doctors and patients
- it may be possible to apply interventions from primary care to reduce non-attendance.

Are these the most important findings?

Are they justified by the evidence presented?

Are they useful?

### Practical activities

By now you should be in a position to evaluate this paper using the same framework as in previous chapters in the book, but hopefully in more detail and with more confidence.

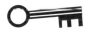 ### Key points

By the end of this chapter, you should be able to:

1 Understand what is meant by a randomised control trial.
2 Critique a published account of a randomised control trial.
3 Read, understand and construct a trial profile.

# 8

# Surveys and questionnaire design

## Introduction

Surveys are widely used (and abused!) in health research. They vary widely in their usage in quantitative and qualitative studies. To consider the wide range of usage of surveys, read the following articles:

- Salisbury C (1997) Postal survey of patients' satisfaction with a general practice out of hours cooperative. *BMJ*. **314**: 1594.
- Cohen G, Forbes J and Garraway M (1996) Can different patient satisfaction survey methods yield consistent results? Comparison of three surveys. *BMJ*. **313**: 841–4.
- Bland JM and Altman DG (1997) Statistics notes: Cronbach's alpha. *BMJ*. **314**: 572.
- Paterson C (1996) Measuring outcomes in primary care: a patient generated measure, MYMOP, compared with the SF-36 health survey. *BMJ*. **312**: 1016–20.

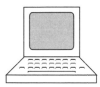

**On-line resource**
You can access these papers via the Chapter 8 section of the website. Alternatively, you may like to go straight to:

http://www.bmj.com

# Questionnaire survey design

The process of survey design is similar to other research processes, so the following stages should look familiar.

## Hypotheses and variables

A hypothesis can be described as 'a tentative answer to a research question' or a 'provisional prediction'. Hypotheses should be:

- stated clearly, using appropriate terminology
- testable
- a statement of relationships between variables
- limited in scope.

## Examples of hypotheses

- Health education programmes influence the number of people who smoke.
- Newspapers affect people's voting patterns.
- Attendance at lectures influences exam marks.
- Diet influences intelligence.

In the above examples, 'something' (e.g. diet, lecture attendance) affects 'something else' (e.g. intelligence, exam marks). These are *variables*. A variable is anything which is free to vary, and in order to describe them *quantitatively*, they have to be expressed in appropriate units (e.g. IQ scores, exam percentages).

| Stage | Description |
|---|---|
| Selecting a topic | The scale of topic should be manageable and not too wide |
| Formulating your hypothesis | The hypothesis or hypotheses should be precise and testable |
| Literature search | What have other people written about this topic? |
| Discussion with 'informants and interested parties' | Are there any people that you will need to speak to in order to clarify issues surrounding this topic? |
| Sampling | Selecting the people to be approached (we shall consider this topic in more detail in Chapter 9) |
| Questionnaire design | Translating the broad objectives of the study into questions that will obtain the necessary information |
| Fieldwork | Collection of data through questionnaire or interview |
| Data processing | Coding and inputting the responses |
| Statistical analysis | Analysing the data |
| Assembly of results | Collating the results |
| Writing up the results | Drawing conclusions/interpretations and relating the findings to other research |

The *pairs* of variables in the above examples have separate names. The variable we manipulate is called the *independent variable* (IV). The variable we are hypothesising which will alter as a result of our manipulations is called the *dependent variable* (DV). The dependent variable alters as a consequence of the value of the independent variable – its value is *dependent* on this. The value of the independent variable is free to vary according to the whims of the experimenters.

| Independent variable | Dependent variable |
| --- | --- |
| • Health education programmes<br>• Newspaper<br>• Attendance at screening programme<br>• Diet | • Number of people who smoke<br>• Voting patterns<br>• Illness<br>• Intelligence |

In practice, many variables can be *either* dependent *or* independent, within the context of a particular study. For example, it could be argued that 'intelligence influences diet' or 'exam marks influence attendance at lectures'.

## Directional hypotheses

In the examples above, words like 'influence' or 'affects' are used without indicating direction. When a hypothesis states a predicted outcome (using words such as reduce, increase, lower, raise), it is called a directional or one-tailed hypothesis. Vaguer types of hypotheses (such as the ones given earlier) are known as non-directional or two-tailed hypotheses.

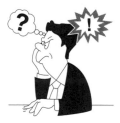

**Questions to think about**

For each of the following subjects:

• the reasons why patients attend clinics
• alternative therapies
• completing prescribed drug programmes
• choice of registered GP.

1  First, write a non-directional (or two-tailed) hypothesis.
2  Now turn the above hypothesis into a directional (or one-tailed) hypothesis.
3  In your hypothesis above, which is the independent variable and which is the dependent variable?

There are two types of questions:

• closed-ended questions
• open-ended questions.

As the names suggest:

- *Closed-ended questions* are designed to allow only a finite set of responses.
- *Open-ended questions* are designed to provide a much wider range of responses.

| Examples of closed-ended questions | | |
| --- | --- | --- |
| *Name* | *Description* | *Example* |
| Dichotomous | Question offering two choices | Did you consult NHS Direct in the last six months? Yes/No |
| Multiple | Question offering three or more choices | Which of these surgery times do you prefer? Morning/Afternoon/Evening |
| Likert scale | Statement with which respondent shows the amount of agreement/ disagreement | I prefer to have injections administered by a nurse rather than a doctor: Strongly agree/Agree/Neither agree nor disagree/Disagree /Strongly disagree |
| Semantic differential | Scale is inscribed between two bipolar words and respondent selects the point that most represents the direction and intensity of their feelings | I find a visit to hospital: Scary ___/___ /___/___/ ___/ Exciting |
| Rank order | Respondent is asked to rate or rank each option that applies | Please indicate in rank order the importance of the following service to you:<br>• Seeing a known doctor outside normal hours<br>• Having a doctor available for home visits<br>• Having telephone advice available<br>• Having service free |
| Numeric | Respondent specifies a particular value | How far (to the nearest kilometre) do you live from your registered GP? |

| Examples of open-ended questions | | |
|---|---|---|
| *Name* | *Description* | *Example* |
| Unstructured | Question that respondents can answer in an unlimited number of ways | Why did you resume smoking? |
| Word association | Words are presented one at a time and respondents give the first word that comes to mind | What is the first thing that comes to mind when you hear the following?<br>• Doctor<br>• Nurse<br>• Receptionist<br>• Consultant |
| Sentence completion | Incomplete sentences are presented, one at a time, and respondents are asked to complete the sentence | My worst experience of the NHS happened when . . . . . . . . . . . . . . . |
| Story completion | An incomplete story is presented and respondents are asked to complete the story | I sat down in the waiting room, picked up a magazine, then looked at the other patients waiting in the room with me . . . . . . . . . . . . . . . . . . . . . . . .<br><br>*now complete the story* |

| *Advantages of closed-ended questions* | *Advantages of open-ended questions* |
|---|---|
| • Quick to answer<br>• Easy to code<br>• No difference between articulate and inarticulate respondents | • Greater freedom of expression<br>• No bias due to limited response ranges<br>• Respondent can qualify their answers |

| *Disadvantages of closed-ended questions* | *Disadvantages of open-ended questions* |
|---|---|
| • Can draw misleading conclusions because of limited range of options<br>• Researcher/interviewer cannot deal with qualifications to responses, e.g. 'Yes, but . . .' or 'It depends', where only Yes/No are given as options | • Time consuming to code<br>• Researcher/interviewer may misinterpret (and therefore misclassify) a response |

Instructions to respondents can have a crucial effect upon response rates:

- Indicate who you are and the purpose of the study.
- Address issues of confidentiality and/or anonymity. You could, for example, include a sentence at the beginning such as, 'All of the information you give me will be treated as completely confidential and it will not be possible for anyone to identify the information you give me when I report my findings'.
- Indicate how the person was selected to receive the questionnaire.
- Indicate how it is to be answered. For example, 'Please answer all of the questions which apply, and leave the remainder blank'.
- Return questions (if not being delivered in person).
- Ensure that each question (or block of similar questions) has a clear instruction on how to respond.
- Indicate the form of the answer (numeric, tick-box, rank, etc.) and how many answers are expected, such as 'most relevant', 'one only' or 'all which apply'.
- Where respondents' answers to an earlier question affects subsequent sets of questions, ensure that the route which they should take is clearly specified. For example, 'If YES, please go to Question 15'.

Other issues to consider are as follows:

- Your respondents may refuse to co-operate if your survey begins with awkward or embarrassing questions.
- People are more likely to give honest replies to personal questions if some *rapport* has been developed with the interviewer. Patients are often sympathetic to surveys from clinicians.
- For the above reasons, it is generally best to keep all questions dealing with demographic information (such as age) at the *end* of the questionnaire.
- Print at the best quality available, people have high expectations of presentation these days.
- Allow adequate space between questions so that you can write down any comments made (but don't waste *too* much paper!!).
- Write the questions themselves in lower case (i.e. like this writing), INSTRUCTIONS IN UPPER CASE (i.e. capital letters).

## *Problem questions*

Some types of questions cause particular problems:

- *Hypothetical questions* A hypothetical question is one in which you are asking respondents to indicate what they *think* they would do under particular imaginary circumstances. These can't always be avoided in some attitudinal research, but they are difficult to administer and often give rise to unreliable answers.
- *Presuming/leading questions* These are often included in poor questionnaires because the researcher feels strongly about a topic and assumes that everyone will be of the same opinion.

- *Questions which rely on memory* Problems which tax the respondent's memory too much are likely to lead to non-response or inaccurate replies. For example, 'What did you have for lunch each day last week?'
- *Questions requiring prior knowledge* For example, 'What is your National Health Service number?'.
- *Mutually exclusive responses* You should always watch out for questions where the multiple choice answers are not mutually exclusive and where a respondent will be uncertain about which category he/she falls under. It seems to be a particular problem with age brackets, and you can often see examples of mistakes here, even in professionally produced surveys.
- *Long questions* If your questions are too long and detailed, the respondent may get lost and the responses will relate only to the beginning or the end of the question.

Before you pilot your questionnaire try going through the checklist opposite to spot whether any of these common mistakes apply to your own questionnaire:

## Piloting your questionnaire

Before you deliver any questionnaire, you should 'pilot' it (i.e. test it) to check that it is going to function effectively. There are a number of reasons why it is important to pilot a questionnaire:

- to test how long it takes to complete
- to check that the questions are not ambiguous
- to check that the instructions are clear
- to allow you to eliminate questions that do not yield usable data.

Ideally it should be piloted on a group similar to the one that will form the population of your study. It is difficult to give an exact number for the pilot group, but as a rule of thumb, try to pilot on about 5–100 of your final sample number. However, the results from the pilot study should not be included with your final results.

If respondents omit certain questions, you should be able to find out why.

Ask the pilot group the following questions:

- How long did it take to complete?
- Were the instructions clear?
- Were any questions unclear or ambiguous?
- Did you object to answering any questions?
- Was the layout clear and attractive?
- Any other comments?

You should then alter your questionnaire to take account of comments made in the pilot study.

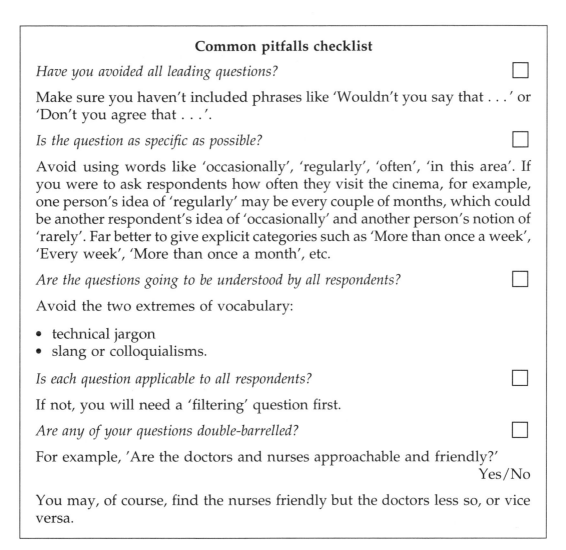

**Common pitfalls checklist**

*Have you avoided all leading questions?*   ☐

Make sure you haven't included phrases like 'Wouldn't you say that . . .' or 'Don't you agree that . . .'.

*Is the question as specific as possible?*   ☐

Avoid using words like 'occasionally', 'regularly', 'often', 'in this area'. If you were to ask respondents how often they visit the cinema, for example, one person's idea of 'regularly' may be every couple of months, which could be another respondent's idea of 'occasionally' and another person's notion of 'rarely'. Far better to give explicit categories such as 'More than once a week', 'Every week', 'More than once a month', etc.

*Are the questions going to be understood by all respondents?*   ☐

Avoid the two extremes of vocabulary:

- technical jargon
- slang or colloquialisms.

*Is each question applicable to all respondents?*   ☐

If not, you will need a 'filtering' question first.

*Are any of your questions double-barrelled?*   ☐

For example, 'Are the doctors and nurses approachable and friendly?'
Yes/No

You may, of course, find the nurses friendly but the doctors less so, or vice versa.

## *Analysis of survey data*

The analysis is determined by the number of variables being examined:

- *Univariate analysis* = one variable (e.g. gender, age). Methods: charts (e.g. bar chart, pie chart) or frequency table.
- *Bivariate analysis* = two variables (e.g. gender + attendance at clinic). Methods: cross-tabulations; scatterplots; regression; comparison of means.
- *Multivariate analysis* = three or more variables (e.g. health behaviours influenced by both education level and gender).

We may define four levels of measurement:

- *Nominal scales* sometimes called 'categorical'. Numbers used to classify things, with no implication that one number is better than another, e.g. hotel rooms, footballers' jerseys, house numbers. They don't have to involve numbers, e.g. blood groups (A, B, O, etc.).
- *Ordinal scales* Involves ordering or ranking of the variable under consideration, e.g. Registrar General Classification of Occupations (I, II, IIN, IIIM, etc.). Categories are ordered with respect to the degree to which they possess particular characteristics without being able to say how much of the characteristic they possess.
- *Interval scales* Not only rank objects by the degree with which they possess a characteristic, but also indicate the exact distance between them. Arithmetic operations can be carried out meaningfully (but cross-scale comparisons are difficult because zero point is not the same).
- *Ratio scales* Like interval scale but with absolute zero (i.e. 'absolutely nothing' there). Examples = physical measurements (length, weight, etc.). Equal intervals are equivalent (e.g. 44 cm is twice as long as 22 cm; unit increase in weight from 12 kg to 18 kg = same as increase in 155 kg to 161 kg).

We may analyse our responses in terms of descriptive or inferential statistics.

- *Descriptive statistics* Summarise patterns in responses (e.g. average age of respondents or number of respondents who buy a product).
- *Inferential statistics* Provide an idea about whether the patterns described in the sample are likely to apply in the population from which the sample is drawn ('tests of significance').

We shall consider data analysis in more detail in Chapter 10.

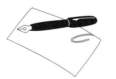

**Practical activities**

Use the framework identified in the Introduction to evaluate the following paper:

- McKinley RK, Manku-Scott T, Hastings AM *et al.* (1997) Reliability and validity of a new measure of patient satisfaction with out of hours primary medical care in the United Kingdom: development of a patient questionnaire. *BMJ.* **314**: 193.

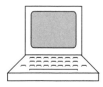

**On-line resource**
You can access this paper via the Chapter 8 section of the website. Alternatively, you may like to go straight to:

http://www.bmj.com

You will find Acrobat and Word 97 versions of the evaluation grid on the website.

**Key points**

By the end of this chapter, you should be able to:

1   Develop a survey appropriate to the needs of a specific problem.
2   Design a survey to minimise bias and maximise its effectiveness.
3   Evaluate reports of surveys by other authors.

# 9

# Sampling, validity and bias

## Introduction

As an introduction to this chapter, please read Chapters 1 to 3 of the following text:

• Coggon D, Rose G and Barker DJP (1997) *Epidemiology for the Uninitiated*. BMJ Books, London.

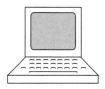

**On-line resource**
You can access this book via the Chapter 9 section of the website. Alternatively, you may like to go straight to:

http://www.bmj.com

or go to the books section of the virtual library.

## Sampling

When undertaking any survey, it is essential that you obtain data from people that are as representative as possible of the group that you are studying. Even with the perfect questionnaire (if such a thing exists), your survey data will only be regarded as useful if it is considered that your respondents are typical of the population as a whole. For this reason, an awareness of the principles of sampling is essential to the implementation of most methods of research, both quantitative and qualitative.

---

**Some key definitions**

| | |
|---|---|
| *Population* | The group of people, items or units under investigation. |
| *Census* | Obtained by collecting information about each and every member of a population. |
| *Sample* | Obtained by collecting information only about some members of a population. |
| *Sampling frame* | The list of people from which the sample is taken. It should be comprehensive, complete and up to date. Examples of sampling frames include electoral registers, postcode address files, telephone directories, and age–sex registers. |

---

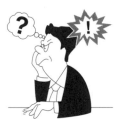

**Questions to think about**

1  If you wanted to deliver a questionnaire to the patients in a primary care group (PCG), would a 'Census' be feasible?
2  If you were undertaking a sample survey of these same patients, what could be your *sampling frame*?

## Probability and non-probability sampling

A probability sample is one in which each member of the population has an equal chance of being selected.

In a non-probability sample, some people have a greater, but unknown, chance than others of selection.

## Probability samples

There are five main types of probability sample as follows:

- simple random sample
- systematic sampling
- random route sampling
- stratified sampling
- multi-stage cluster sampling.

Each has its advantages and disadvantages. The choice of which to use depends on:

- the nature of research problem
- the availability of a good sampling frame
- money available
- time available
- the desired level of accuracy in the sample and data collection methods.

The five methods are summarised below.

---

### Simple random sample

| *Procedure* | *Characteristics* |
|---|---|
| • Obtain a complete sampling frame | • Each person has same chance as any other of being selected |
| • Give each case a unique number, starting at one | • Standard against which other methods are sometimes evaluated |
| • Decide on the required sample size | • Suitable where population is relatively small and where sampling frame is complete and up to date |
| • Select that many numbers from a table of random numbers or using a computer | |
| • Decide on a pattern of movement through the table and stick to it, e.g. numbers from every second column and every row | |

| *Advantages* | *Disadvantages* |
|---|---|
| • Each person has same chance as any other of being selected | • Only suitable where population is relatively small |
| | • Requires complete and up to date sampling frame |

### Systematic sampling

| *Procedure* | *Characteristics* |
|---|---|
| • Obtain a complete sampling frame | • Each person has same chance as any other of being selected |
| • Give each case a unique number, starting at one | • Suitable where population is relatively small and where sampling frame is complete and up to date |
| • Decide on the required sample size | |

- Work out *sampling fraction* by dividing population size by required sample size, e.g. for a population of 500 and a sample of 100, the sampling fraction is 1/5, i.e. you will select one person out of every five in the population. Random number needs to be used only to decide on starting point
- Move through list (sample frame) picking every nth name

|          *Advantages*          |          *Disadvantages*          |
| --- | --- |
| • Each person has same chance as any other of being selected | • Only suitable where population is relatively small<br>• Requires complete and up to date sampling frame<br>• The disadvantage of this approach is the effect of periodicity, i.e. bias caused by particular characteristics arising in the sampling frame at regular units* |

* An example of this would occur if you used a sampling frame of adult residents in an area composed predominantly of couples or young families. If this list was arranged: husband/wife/husband/wife, etc. and if every tenth person was to be interviewed, there would be an increased chance of males being selected.

## Random route sampling

### Procedure

- Obtain a complete sampling frame, usually electoral register
- The address is selected at random from sampling frame as a starting point
- The interviewer is then given instructions to identify further addresses by taking alternate left- and right-hand turns at road junctions and calling at every nth address (shop, garage, etc.)

### Characteristics

- Used in market research surveys – mainly for sampling households, shops, garages and other premises in urban areas

### Advantages

- May be time saving
- Bias may be reduced because interviewer has to call at clearly defined addresses – not able to choose

### Disadvantages

- Requires complete and up to date sampling frame
- Characteristics of particular areas (e.g. poor/rich) may mean that sample is not representative
- Open to abuse by interviewer because difficult to check that instructions fully carried out

## Stratified sampling

*Procedure*

- All people in sampling frame are divided into 'strata' (groups or categories)
- Within each stratum, a simple random sample or systematic sample is selected as described

*Characteristics*

- To ensure that a sample of 50 patients from a group of 500 contains both male and female patients in the same proportions as in the full 500, that population is first divided into male and female. In this case, there are 220 male patients and 280 females, therefore our sample becomes 22 males and 28 females
- These would be selected using simple random or systematic sample methods

*Advantages*

- Designed to ensure sample reflects overall population mix

*Disadvantages*

- Requires complete and up to date sampling frame
- Extra complexity in design
- Choice of groups may reflect researcher's bias

## Multi-stage cluster sampling

*Procedure*

- First draw sample of areas
- Initially large areas selected then progressively smaller areas within larger area are sampled
- Eventually end up with sample of households and use one of the above methods of selecting individuals from these selected households

*Characteristics*

- Designed to minimise cost of final interviewing

*Advantages*

- Cost of final interviewing is minimised
- Suitable for larger populations

*Disadvantages*

- Requires complete and up to date sampling frame
- Extra complexity in design

## Non-probability samples

It is not always possible to undertake a probability method of sampling, such as in random sampling. For example, there is not a complete sampling frame available for certain groups of the population, such as the elderly; people who are attending a football match; people who shop in a particular part of town. Another factor to bear in mind is that many of the probability sampling methods described above may mean that researchers would have to undertake a postal or telephone survey delivery or might be expected to go from house to house. A probability sample with a poor response rate does not in the end give you a particularly good representation of the population being examined.

Non-probability methods have the following advantages:

- they are cheaper
- they may be used when sampling frame is not available
- they are useful when the population is so widely dispersed that cluster sampling would not be efficient
- they are often used in exploratory studies, e.g. for hypothesis generation.

Some research is not interested in working out what proportion of population gives a particular response, but rather in obtaining a picture of the range of responses on ideas that people have.

Non-probability methods include:

- *Purposive sampling* A purposive sample is one that is selected by the researcher subjectively. The researcher attempts to obtain a sample that appears to him/her to be representative of the population and will usually try to ensure that a range from one extreme to the other is included. This method has often been used in political polling where districts are chosen because their pattern has in the past provided a good idea of outcomes for the whole electorate.
- *Quota sampling* Quota sampling is often used in market research. Interviewers are required to find cases with particular characteristics. They are given quota of particular types of people to interview and the quota are organised so that the final sample should be representative of the population. The disadvantage of quota sampling is that interviewers choose who they like within the specified criteria and may therefore select those who are easiest to interview, so bias can result. Also, it is impossible to estimate accuracy because this is not a random sample.
- *Convenience sampling* A convenience sample is used when you simply stop anybody in the street who is prepared to stop, or when you wander round a business, a shop, a restaurant or a theatre, asking people you meet whether they will answer your questions. Within a general practice, this might be those patients who attended for an appointment on a particular day. In other words, the sample comprises subjects who are simply available in a convenient way to

the researcher. There is no randomness and the likelihood of bias is high. You can't draw any meaningful conclusions from the results you obtain.

However, this method is often the only feasible one, particularly for those with restricted time and resources, and can legitimately be used provided its limitations are clearly understood and stated.

- *Snowball sampling* With this approach, you initially contact a few potential respondents and then ask them whether they know of anybody with the same characteristics that you are looking for in your research. For example, if you wanted to interview a sample of patients with a particular disability your initial contacts may well have knowledge through a support group of others with the same disability.
- *Self-selection* Self-selection is perhaps self-explanatory. Respondents themselves decide that they would like to take part in your survey.

## Non-responses

You will always have to take account of non-responses. Health surveys are generally better received than those for market research purposes, but you will still have to deal with:

- those who refuse
- those who are uncontactable
- those who are uninterviewable.

This can cause you two major problems. The most obvious is an unacceptable reduction in sample size. Equally important can be the introduction of bias if your non-responses are not completely random, for example if there are gender differences in the response rates. Remember men aged 18–50 are notorious for ignoring their health!

## Sample size

The sample size you will need depends upon:

- the size of the effect that you are looking for
- the sampling methodology used.

Because of the complexity of this issue, I suggest that you find a tame statistician to help with this thorny issue if you are inspired to do your own work. If you are reading a study by someone else, then ask yourself the following questions:

> **Sample size checklist when reading studies**
>
> 1  Does the article justify the sample size used?
> 2  Does the article justify the sampling methodology used?
> 3  Does the article say what response rate was achieved?
> 4  Does the article indicate what response rate was anticipated?
> 5  Does the article suggest what steps were taken to minimise bias in the sample?
> 6  Are there any obvious biases that are not mentioned?

# Bias and validity

Now read Chapter 4 of the following text:

• Coggon D, Rose G and Barker DJP (1997) *Epidemiology for the Uninitiated*. BMJ Books, London.

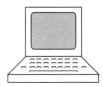

**On-line resource**
You can access this book via the Chapter 9 section of the website. Alternatively, you may like to go straight to:

http://www.bmj.com

or go to the books section of the virtual library.

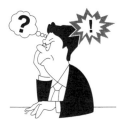

**Questions to think about**

In this chapter, we have focused upon surveys, whilst the treatment presented in *Epidemiology for the Uninitiated* is oriented more towards a clinical perspective.

1  What similarities do you observe between the approaches?
2  What differences do you observe between the approaches?
3  What differences do you observe in their view of the problem of bias?

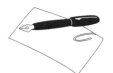

## Practical activities

Use the framework identified in the Introduction to evaluate the following paper:

• Maheux B, Haley N, Rivard M and Gervais A (1999) Do physicians assess lifestyle health risks during general medical examinations? A survey of general practitioners and obstetrician-gynaecologists in Quebec. *CMAJ.* **160**: 1830.

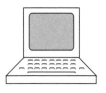

### On-line resource
You can access this paper via the Chapter 9 section of the website.

You will find Acrobat and Word 97 versions of the evaluation grid on the website.

### Key points

By the end of this chapter, you should be able to:

1   Develop a sampling strategy for a study.
2   Evaluate reports of sampling strategies by other authors.
3   Compare and contrast different approaches to sampling.

**10**

# Analysing your data

## Introduction

By now you must have been expecting more x's and y's, perhaps even a few $\Sigma$ and $\Theta$s to contend with. The short answer is that there is not room in a book this size to deal with the whole gamut of statistics. For this kind of information, please look at the list of resources at the end of the chapter to help with statistics where you will find books, CD-ROMs and an on-line statistics course. I strongly encourage you to do so!

In this chapter we will introduce the principles and help you interpret some of the figures that appear in published articles. We shall use a published article to consider the use of statistical techniques.

## What do all the statistics mean?

In this chapter we shall use the following paper as a teaching aid:

- Emanuel EJ, Fairclough DL, Slutsman J *et al.* (1999) Assistance from family members, friends, paid care givers, and volunteers in the care of terminally ill patients. *NEJM.* **341**: 956–63.

**On-line resource**
You can access this paper via the Chapter 10 section of the website.

In order to do this you will need to register for the on-line version of the *New England Journal of Medicine*. This is free and gives you access to all research articles older than six months prior to today. Seems like a reasonable deal to me.

The paper was concerned with the assistance given to terminally ill patients. We shall use extracts from the paper to show how statistics are used and hopefully what they mean. We shall consider the results section. The opening sentence is as follows:

*The mean age of the 988 terminally ill patients we interviewed was 66.5 years; 59.4 percent were 65 or older (Table 1). Men were significantly more likely than women to be married or living with a partner (74.4 percent vs 45.9 percent, P < 0.001); 64.8 percent of white patients, 45.2 percent of Hispanic patients, and 37.0 percent of black patients reported being married or living with a partner (P = 0.001 for the overall comparison).*

Table 1 from the paper is reproduced opposite:

**Table 1** Characteristics of the terminally ill patients in the study, the US population in 1997, and the subjects in the study to understand prognoses and preferences for outcomes and risks of treatment (SUPPORT)*

| Characteristic | Total | | | Age ≥ 65 years | | |
|---|---|---|---|---|---|---|
| | Study patients (N = 988) | US population 198 107 000 | SUPPORT subjects (N = 9105) | Study patients (N = 587) | US population 34 076 000 | SUPPORT subjects (N = 4513) |
| | *Percentage* | | | | | |
| Sex | | | | | | |
| Male | 48.5 | 48.2 | 43.7 | 53.5 | 41.1 | 54.6 |
| Female | 51.5 | 51.9 | 56.3 | 46.5 | 58.9 | 45.4 |
| Race or ethnic group | | | | | | |
| White | 78.9 | 75.2 | 79.4 | 82.5 | 84.7 | 85.0 |
| Black | 13.7 | 11.2 | 15.3 | 12.6 | 8.0 | 12.0 |
| Hispanic | 3.2 | 9.6 | 3.2 | 1.7 | 4.9 | 1.6 |
| Other | 4.2 | 4.1 | 2.1 | 3.1 | 2.4 | 1.4 |
| Education | | | | | | |
| Eighth grade or less | 14.0 | 7.2 | 16.4 | 20.4 | 18.8 | 22.7 |
| Some high school | 18.9 | 11.4 | 28.1 | 19.8 | 15.7 | 27.6 |
| High-school graduate | 27.4 | 33.4 | 27.7 | 24.6 | 34.3 | 25.4 |
| Some college | 21.8 | 19.4 | 15.8 | 17.2 | 12.9 | 13.3 |
| College graduate | 11.5 | 21.7 | 6.8 | 11.2 | 12.9 | 6.3 |
| Graduate training | 6.3 | 6.9 | 5.2 | 6.7 | 5.4 | 4.7 |
| Religion | | | | | | |
| Protestant | 61.8 | 58.0 | 52.0 | 61.8 | NA | 48.4 |
| Catholic | 25.4 | 25.0 | 27.9 | 25.3 | NA | 28.8 |
| Jewish | 4.3 | 2.0 | 8.5 | 5.0 | NA | 13.1 |
| Other | 8.4 | 15.0 | 11.7 | 8.0 | NA | 9.7 |
| Household income† | | | | | | |
| < $15 000 | 38.4 | 20.3 | 55.9 | 41.9 | 37.8 | 62.4 |
| $15 000–$24 999 | 21.1 | 15.4 | 20.5 | 23.1 | 23.4 | 23.1 |
| $25 000–$49 999 | 24.9 | 30.0 | 15.2 | 23.6 | 24.7 | 9.0 |
| ≥ $50 000 | 15.6 | 34.3 | 8.4 | 11.4 | 14.1 | 5.4 |
| Marital status | | | | | | |
| Married | 59.7 | 59.6 | 53.4 | 57.4 | 55.6 | 52.2 |
| Widowed | 20.3 | 7.0 | 20.1 | 29.6 | 33.4 | 32.9 |
| Divorced | 9.0 | 9.9 | 15.2 | 4.9 | 6.8 | 9.7 |
| Other | 10.8 | 23.5 | 11.4 | 8.1 | 4.2 | 6.1 |

*Participants in our study were 22 to 109 years of age; the figures for the US population in 1997 include only persons older than 18 years, except for the figures for level of education, which included only persons older than 25 years. Because of rounding, percentages may not total 100. Data on US population are from the Bureau of Census. Data on SUPPORT subjects are from Russell Phillips and Jane Soukup (personal communication). NA denotes not available.

† In SUPPORT, income is recorded as under $11 000 and $11 000 to $25 000. Consequently, the categories do not precisely match the data from our study or the Census data.

In this opening paragraph, we have illustrated the two major types of statistics employed. The first type is *descriptive* statistics, used to describe the age distribution:

· *The mean age of the 988 terminally ill patients we interviewed was 66.5 years.*

In practice, to describe a dataset fully we need to define three things:

• a measure of centre
• a measure of spread or dispersion
• an indication of the shape of the distribution.

For large populations, we generally assume that natural factors such as age, height, weight would follow a normal distribution. This means that they have the commonly occurring 'bell' shape (*see* Figure 10.1).

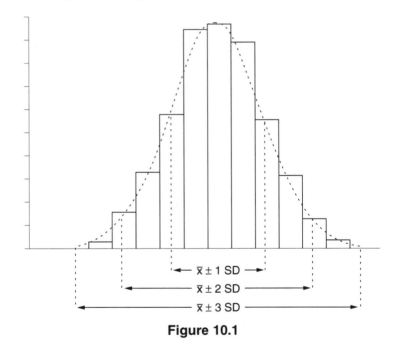

**Figure 10.1**

A normal distribution has the characteristic that the three most common measures of centre are the same:

• *the arithmetic mean*, the total divided by the number of data points
• *the median*, the middle value if the data is arranged in rank order
• *the mode*, the most common value.

It is also symmetrical, expressed mathematically as a skewedness of zero. In practice, many of the commonly used statistical techniques assume that the data shows a normal distribution.

Once we know where the centre is, and that its shape is normal, then the final parameter needed to define it is its dispersion or spread. This is generally measured as its standard deviation. For a normal distribution, approximately 68% of the values lie within 1 standard deviation of the mean.

In practice, in the study described, this population is a skewed sample in terms of age because the people are all selected by their condition.

The next statement compares two data sets and quotes a figure:

*Men were significantly more likely than women to be married or living with a partner (74.4 percent vs 45.9 percent, P < 0.001).*

This looks simple; but it has a number of key elements. The first is the word 'significant'. This refers to statistical significance, not clinical significance. It indicates that the p-value is less than 0.05. This is confirmed by the figure at the end of the sentence. The sentence tells us that 74% of men were married or living with a partner, compared with 46% of women.

To explore further the meaning of significance, we need to extract the raw data from Table 1:

|  | *Male* | *Female* | **Total** |
|---|---|---|---|
| 'Married' | 357 | 234 | 591 |
| 'Single' | 122 | 275 | 397 |
| **Total** | 479 | 509 | 988 |

---

### Explanation

We know that of 988 people in the study, 48.5% are male, corresponding to 479, and 51.5% are female corresponding to 509. Of the males, we know that 74.4% (357) are married or living with a partner, and that 45.9% of the females are married or living with a partner.

---

In order to calculate whether this is a significant difference, we then use a chi-squared test. In this test, we set up something called the null hypothesis. This is the hypothesis that there is no association between marital status and gender. The test examines the probability or likelihood that this null hypothesis is true. If the probability that the null hypothesis is true is very low, then that provides evidence that the opposite, i.e that there is an association, is true.

To calculate this we first work out how many married males we would expect if there was no association. This is a matter of simple ratio. If there is no association we expect the number of married males to be:

Proportion of married people in the general population

$\times$ the number of males in the population.

For our example, this becomes:

$$\frac{591}{988} \times 479 = 286.$$

Similarly for the married females, if there is no association, we expect the number to be given by:

Proportion of married people in the general population

$\times$ the number of females in the population.

For our example, this becomes:

$$\frac{591}{988} \times 509 = 304.$$

For the single men, if there is no association, we expect the number to be given by:

Proportion of single people in the general population

$\times$ the number of males in the population.

For our example, this becomes:

$$\frac{397}{988} \times 479 = 193$$

And finally, for the single women, if there is no association, we expect the number to be given by:

Proportion of single people in the general population

$\times$ the number of females in the population.

For our example, this becomes:

$$\frac{397}{988} \times 509 = 205$$

This gives us what we call our expected values table:

|  | Male | Female | Total |
|---|---|---|---|
| 'Married' | 286 | 304 | 591 |
| 'Single' | 193 | 205 | 397 |
| **Total** | 479 | 509 | 988 |

In comparing these tables, we can use a computer to calculate the probability that the null hypothesis is true (*see* pages 80–1 for further details).

Excel gives the p-value as **5.04455E-20**, or $5 \times 10^{-20}$ which is certainly very small, and less than 0.001, as quoted in the article.

Traditionally, researchers have taken a value of less than 0.05 as statistically significant. However, there is a current trend for quoting the confidence interval as well. Confidence intervals may be applied to almost any statistical test including means. Note that the above descriptive analysis does not include a 95% confidence limit for the mean.

Our study relates to a sample of the population. Therefore if we took a different sample, we might expect to get a different answer, and our answer can only be an estimate. How good an estimate will depend upon:

• the size of the sample; the bigger our sample, the more confidence we can have in the answer.
• the variation within the population; the more uniform the population, the more we can have confidence that our sample will reflect the whole.

Traditionally confidence limits are quoted to 95%, i.e. the range of p-values (in our case) within which we may be 95% sure that the true value lies. Clearly, if the entire range of p-values defined by the 95% confidence limits lies below 0.05, then we may say that we have 95% confidence that the association is significant.

To find out how to calculate this in practice, refer to the tools section on pages 80–1.

We shall merely note that this paper does not quote confidence limits for its p-values, which means that we cannot know how representative the calculated p-values of the general population are.

In practice, with a relatively large sample size and a very significant p-value, it seems unlikely that there would be a problem.

In practice, this basic approach is repeated throughout the paper. In reality, the test results presented are incomplete from a statistical perspective; the mean lacking any measure of dispersion or confidence. Similarly, the p-values quoted do not have any confidence limits. The reality is that many published studies lack this kind of data, but get away with it by bamboozling the reader with an impressive range of p-values, etc.

The need for this kind of measure goes back to our discussion of scientific method earlier in the book. In healthcare trials, we are not dealing with controlled scientific experiments. Rather we are dealing with situations where we seek to randomise out extraneous factors and therefore deal in probabilities.

# Tools for data analysis

There are three computer tools for data analysis that I have used in my own work.

## *Epi Info*

Epi Info was produced by the World Health Organization for epidemiologists. In today's world, it may best be described as quirky. Its major drawback is that it runs in DOS, which for those readers under 25, is the old style text-based operating system that all PCs used until Windows was introduced.

The advantages of Epi Info are:

- it has a powerful analysis section, which readily produces good results
- it does produce error messages or uses different algorithms to produce best results, e.g. with small samples
- it quotes overtly all the algorithms and sources thereof
- it does not use a mouse which lends itself to use on a laptop
- it runs on PCs of limited power which encourages its use in developing countries
- it is in the public domain, so is free.

In reality, I like Epi Info but it has as much street credibility as a Lada car. Its graphing facilities are about as attractive. For quick and easy chi-squared tests it is unbeatable.

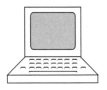

**On-line resource**
You can download Epi Info from the Internet.

You will find the link in the Chapter 10 section of the website.

## *Excel*<sup>TM</sup>

Excel is a very popular programme. Many people have a copy as part of Microsoft Office. Its advantages are:

- standard Windows interface makes it familiar and easy to use for many people
- good graphing facilities
- easy to produce basic descriptive statistics.

Against this:

- many of the more complex functions are either difficult to access or omitted

- the algorithms used are not transparent
- some authors have argued that Excel produces erroneous results for statistical tests such as chi-squared tests.

If you want to use Excel, consider a number of additional resources. The following will help you get the most from Excel in a healthcare context:

- Gillies AC (2001) *Excel for Clinical Governance.* Radcliffe Medical Press, Oxford.

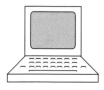

**On-line resource**
You can buy this book on-line.

You will find a link in the statistics resources section of the website.

If you want to use Excel for research for publication, you may also like to consider one of the external add-ins that can be bought, which add reliable and transparent statistical algorithms to Excel. One such application is produced by Iain Buchan at Cambridge University.

## *SPSS*

This is the granddaddy of serious statistical software. If Epi Info has the street credibility of a Lada, this has the credibility of a Lexus or BMW. It has the advantages of:

- serious street credibility
- reliable algorithms
- all the functionality you could ever wish for.

Against this, I find it a little cumbersome in use, and rather bewildering to the beginner. Certainly if you have access to a University or other facility where SPSS is available and there are people to help you use it, then it is probably the package to use.

# More resources

This chapter is very much an introduction. We cannot cover, for example, different techniques used to carry out statistical tests. Therefore, you are strongly encouraged to go on and find out more. Here are some resources I recommend:

- Hart AE (2001) *Making Sense of Statistics in Healthcare.* Radcliffe Medical Press, Oxford.

This is a book. In fact it is *the* book to read about statistics. It is superbly readable and almost devoid of formulae. It explains things that I have never understood. It has a useful glossary of terms at the end of the book. If you buy anything in this section, buy this book.

• Morris S and Szuscikiewicz J (2001) *Statistics for the Terrified, Version 5*. Radcliffe Medical Press, Oxford.

If you prefer a more active learning style try this CD-ROM. It takes you through a lot of statistics in a fun and active learning format.

• Altman DG (1991) *Practical Statistics for Medical Research*. Chapman & Hall, London.

This is a more comprehensive and complex text, but its extensive use of real examples from the literature stops it from becoming turgid. My favourite example is the link between caffeine consumption and marital status!

• Swinscow TDV (1997) *Statistics at Square One*. BMJ Books, London. (Available on-line.)

This is a standard textbook that has been made available on-line. It lacks, in my humble opinion, some of the lightness of touch of some of the other resources cited here. But it is a well-known text.

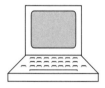

**On-line resource**
You can buy all of these resources on-line, and access the Swinscow text directly.

You will find a link in the statistics resources section of the website.

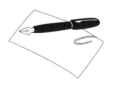

**Practical activities**

Use the framework identified in the Introduction to evaluate the *NEJM* paper, paying particular attention to the use of statistics.

• Emanuel EJ, Fairclough DL, Slutsman J *et al.* (1999) Assistance from family members, friends, paid care givers, and volunteers in the care of terminally ill patients. *NEJM*. **341**: 956–63.

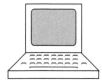

**On-line resource**

You can access this paper via the Chapter 10 section of the website.

In order to do this you will need to register for the on-line version of the *New England Journal of Medicine*. This is free and gives you access to all research articles older than six months prior to today. Seems like a reasonable deal to me.

You will find Acrobat and Word 97 versions of the evaluation grid on the website.

 **Key points**

By the end of this chapter, you should be able to:

1 Read and understand better the statistics used in published studies.
2 Have an intelligent conversation with a statistician about study design.
3 Select a data analysis tool suitable for your needs.

# Part Three
# Methods for qualitative research

# 11

# Overview of qualitative methods in research

## Introduction

Qualitative research is a growth area, especially in primary care. It is interesting to note that all of the studies published to date (at the time of writing) in the *BMJ* using qualitative research have been in the general practice section.

Let us start by considering the following three papers:

- Mays N and Pope C (2000) Qualitative research in healthcare: assessing quality in qualitative research. *BMJ*. **320**: 50–2.
- Pope C, Ziebland S and Mays N (2000) Qualitative research in healthcare: analysing qualitative data. *BMJ*. **320**: 114–16.
- Meyer J (2000) Qualitative research in healthcare: using qualitative methods in health related action research. *BMJ*. **320**: 178–81.

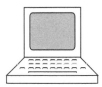

**On-line resource**
You can access these papers via the Chapter 11 section of the website.

# Qualitative research

From this introductory reading, think about the following questions:

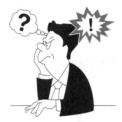

### Questions to think about

1 What specific methods are identified within the papers?
2 What approaches are identified?
3 What advantages are given for this type of research?
4 What disadvantages are given for this type of research?

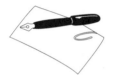

### Practical activities

Record your answers to these questions in a grid like the one below:

| | |
|---|---|
| Specific methods for qualitative research | |
| Approaches to qualitative research | |
| Advantages of qualitative research | |
| Disadvantages of qualitative research | |

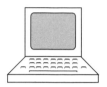

**On-line resource**
You will find Acrobat and Word 97 versions of this grid on the website.

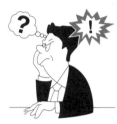

**Questions to think about**

In Part Two, we identified that qualitative research is often regarded as second class, especially in certain sectors. Which groups do you think are likely to be least open to qualitative methods, and why?

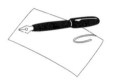

**Practical activities**

1  Use the framework identified in the Introduction to evaluate the following study:

• Gardner K, Chapple A and Green J (1999) Barriers to referral in patients with angina: qualitative study – Commentary: generalisability and validity in qualitative research. *BMJ*. **319**: 418–21.

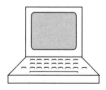

**On-line resource**
You can access this paper via the Chapter 11 section of the website.

You will find Acrobat and Word 97 versions of the evaluation grid on the website.

2  Consider how well this framework addresses papers of a more qualitative perspective.

**Key points**

By the end of this chapter, you should be able to:

1 Describe what qualitative research is.
2 Outline the methods used in qualitative research.
3 Outline the strengths and weaknesses of qualitative approaches.

# 12

# A systematic approach to qualitative research

## Introduction

Read the following paper:

- Greenhalgh T and Taylor R (1997) How to read a paper: papers that go beyond numbers (qualitative research). *BMJ*. **315**: 740–3.

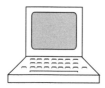

**On-line resource**
You can access this paper via the Chapter 12 section of the website.

## Qualitative research

According to Greenhalgh and Taylor (1997), qualitative research aims to make sense of, or interpret, phenomena in terms of the meanings people bring to them. They identify three characteristics of good qualitative research:

---

### Characteristics of good qualitative research

- Good qualitative research will have a clearly formulated question.
- Good qualitative research will use more than one research method (triangulation).
- Analysis should be done using explicit systematic and reproducible methods.

From Greenhalgh and Taylor (1997)

---

Further, they provide a series of questions that may be used to evaluate qualitative research studies:

---

### Checklist of questions to evaluate qualitative research

1 Was there a clearly formulated question?
2 Was a qualitative approach appropriate?
3 How were the setting and subjects selected?
4 What was the researcher's perspective and has this been taken into account?
5 Methods – are they described in enough detail?
6 Methods – what quality control measures were used?
7 Are the results significant?
8 Conclusions – are they justified?
9 Are the results transferable?

From Greenhalgh and Taylor (1997)

---

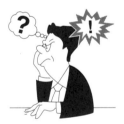 **Questions to think about**

Using the Greenhalgh and Taylor paper, and the paper considered in Chapter 11 – Mays N and Pope C (2000) Qualitative research in healthcare: assessing quality in qualitative research. *BMJ*. **320**: 50–2:

1 Revise the questions used to evaluate papers from an academic perspective to better fit the needs of qualitative research.
2 Consider the other perspectives, do they need to be reconsidered from the perspective of qualitative research?

3   Do the other perspectives contribute to the continued resistance to qualitative research in many healthcare situations?

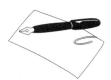

## Practical activities

1   Use your responses to produce a modified evaluation framework suitable for qualitative studies.
2   Use your modified framework to evaluate the following paper:

* Ruston A, Clayton J, Calnan M and Green J (1998) Patients' action during their cardiac event: qualitative study exploring differences and modifiable factors – Commentary: grounded theory and the constant comparative method. *BMJ.* **316**: 1060–5.

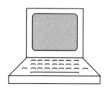

### On-line resource
You can access this paper via the Chapter 12 section of the website.

It is suggested that you produce your own evaluation framework based upon the Word version of the standard template downloadable from the website.

## Key points

By the end of this chapter, you should be able to:

1   Read critically a paper describing a qualitative research study.
2   Identify specific features of qualitative studies requiring particular scrutiny.

# 13

# Design of a qualitative research study

## Introduction

In this chapter, we shall consider the design of a qualitative study through a number of stages:

- the research question
- methods selection
- empirical work and analysis
- evaluation and reflection.

Of these, the third is dealt with in more detail in Chapters 14–16. We shall focus here on the other three, as these are considered generic to qualitative research, indeed to all research.

## The research question

Some authors believe that the sole purpose of qualitative research is to define a research question for 'proper' research, i.e. a randomised controlled trial (RCT).

However, Greenhalgh and Taylor (1997) emphasise the importance of a clear research question for qualitative research (accessible through the Chapter 12 section of the website):

A previous article in this series explained that one of the first things you should look for in any research paper is a statement of why the research was done and what specific question it addressed. *Qualitative papers are no exception to this rule: there is absolutely no scientific value in interviewing or observing people just for the sake of it.* Papers that cannot define their topic of research more closely than, 'We decided to interview 20 patients with epilepsy' inspire little confidence that the researchers really knew what they were studying or why.

You might be more inclined to read on if the paper stated in its introduction something like, 'Epilepsy is a common and potentially disabling condition, and up to 20% of patients do not remain free of fits while taking medication. Anti-epileptic medication is known to have unpleasant side effects, and several studies have shown that a high proportion of patients do not take their tablets regularly. We therefore decided to explore patients' beliefs about epilepsy and their perceived reasons for not taking their medication'.

It may be argued that there is an even greater need for clarity in defining the research question in qualitative studies.

Consider the following introduction to a paper describing a recent qualitative study:

---

Over recent years, communication and information have increasingly been considered important in helping people to cope with cancer. A diagnosis of cancer may invoke uncertainty, fear, and loss that can be alleviated by information. Research has indicated that the vast majority of cancer patients want to be informed about their illness. However, it is also recognised that patients vary in how much information they want and that this may change during their illness. These attitudes are reflected in the efforts that patients make to obtain further information or to resist information that is offered to them. In 1980, Ingelfinger, at that time an oncologist and editor of the *New England Journal of Medicine*, reported that when he discovered he had cancer he did not want all available information nor to have to face the uncertainties of the different treatment choices offered to him. This hints at the complexity of providing information in oncology; information may be ignored or avoided by patients, regardless of their prior knowledge or occupation.

For those who provide care to cancer patients, the challenge is finding a way of providing information that is appropriate for patients who may benefit from knowing something about their illness and its treatment but may not wish to know everything about it at all times. This is particularly important in the light of the Government's current commitment to build on the work of the Calman–Hine Expert Advisory Group to improve cancer care. Recent developments include plans for a national cancer information strategy, the details of which have yet to be agreed. It is likely that such an initiative could include 'core information packages' for all patients (NHS Information Authority, draft consultation document of cancer information strategy).

In light of the move toward more formal provision of information, there is an urgent need to understand the ways that and the reasons why patients may choose not to seek or may resist further information about their cancer. This paper reports the findings of a study that explored patients' reasons for not wanting further information.

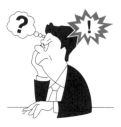

**Questions to think about**

1   Does the introduction describe a specific research question?
2   What is it?

Now read the abstract from the same study:

*Objectives*:  To explore why cancer patients do not want or seek information about their condition beyond that volunteered by their physicians at times during their illness.

*Design*:  Qualitative study based on in-depth interviews.

*Setting*:  Outpatient oncology clinics at a London cancer centre.

*Participants*:  17 patients with cancer diagnosed in previous six months.

*Main outcome measures*:  Analysis of patients' narratives to identify key themes and categories.

*Results*: While all patients wanted basic information on diagnosis and treatment, not all wanted further information at all stages of their illness. Three overarching attitudes to their management of cancer limited patients' desire for and subsequent efforts to obtain further information: faith, hope, and charity. Faith in their doctor's medical expertise precluded the need for patients to seek further information themselves. Hope was essential for patients to carry on with life as normal and could be maintained through silence and avoiding information, especially too detailed or 'unsafe' information. Charity to fellow patients, especially those seen as more needy than themselves, was expressed in the recognition that scarce resources including information and explanations had to be shared and meant that limited information was accepted as inevitable.

*Conclusions*: Cancer patients' attitudes to cancer and their strategies for coping with their illness can constrain their wish for information and their efforts to obtain it. In developing recommendations, the Government's cancer information strategy should attend to variations in patients' desires for information and the reasons for them.

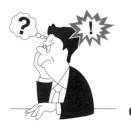

### Questions to think about

1   Does the abstract help describe a specific research question?
2   What is it?

Now read the whole paper:

• Leydon GM *et al*. (2000) Cancer patients' information needs and information seeking behaviour: in-depth interview study. *BMJ*. **320**: 909–13.

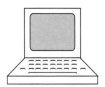

**On-line resource**
You can access this paper via the Chapter 13 section of the website.

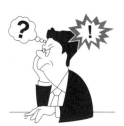

### Questions to think about

1   Now do you see a specific research question?
2   What is it?

The research is described as 'exploratory' in nature. What are the advantages and disadvantages of this type of approach?

# Methods selection

Greenhalgh and Taylor (1997) identify the following types of methods within qualitative research:

---

**Methods for qualitative research**

- *Documents* – Study of documentary accounts of events, such as meetings.
- *Passive observation* – Systematic watching of behaviour and talk in natural occurring settings.
- *Participant observation* – Observation in which the researcher also occupies a role or part in the setting, in addition to observing.
- *In-depth interviews* – Face-to-face conversation with the purpose of exploring issues or topics in detail. Does not use preset questions, but is shaped by a defined set of topics.
- *Focus groups* – Method of group interview which explicitly includes and uses the group interaction to generate data.

From Greenhalgh and Taylor (1997)

---

In quantitative studies, it is usual to define a single research method. Further, we usually have a very hierarchical view of the merits of different approaches, which may be expressed as crudely as 'RCT good, anything else bad'! However, there are many problems that are not well suited to RCTs, and other approaches can offer insight and understanding.

In selecting methods for a qualitative study, the following principles should be borne in mind:

- methods may be determined by the situation under consideration
- even where the situation does not absolutely determine the methods to be used, a desire for minimum disturbance of the situation under scrutiny will be a major factor
- a combination of different methods is desirable. We shall return to this later in the book.

Consider the following study:

---

**Domestic violence and primary care: attitudes, practices, and beliefs**
Sugg NK, Thompson RS, Thompson DC *et al*.

*Objective*: To assess the attitudes and beliefs of the primary care provider team (physicians, physician assistants, nurses, and medical assistants) toward the identification and management of abused patients and perpetrators of domestic violence (DV).

*Design*:

*Setting and subjects*: Five primary care clinics with 240 providers at a large urban health maintenance organisation.

*Results*:

*Conclusions*: This study provides important information about current knowledge, attitudes, and beliefs of healthcare providers toward the diagnosis and management of DV. This information should prove useful to all who attempt to design clinical strategies and educational programs to address this issue.

 **Questions to think about**

1   What methods might you use to investigate this situation?
2   Why?

Now consider the full abstract:

**Domestic violence and primary care: attitudes, practices, and beliefs**
Sugg NK, Thompson RS, Thompson DC *et al.*

*Objective*: To assess the attitudes and beliefs of the primary care provider team (physicians, physician assistants, nurses, and medical assistants) toward the identification and management of abused patients and perpetrators of domestic violence (DV).

*Design*: Survey of the healthcare team using a confidential questionnaire.

*Setting and subjects*: Five primary care clinics with 240 providers at a large urban health maintenance organisation.

*Results*: The response rate was 86% (206 respondents). Fifty percent of clinicians and 70% of nurses/assistants believed that the prevalence of DV in their practice was 1% or less; 1 in 10 clinicians and nearly half of nurses/assistants had never identified an abused person; 45% of clinicians never or seldom asked about DV when examining injured patients; and all participants were much less confident in asking about DV than about smoking or consuming alcohol. Twenty-five percent believed the abused person's personality led to the violence; 28% believed they did not have strategies to help abused persons; and 20% were concerned for their personal safety in discussing DV. Only 10% believed they had management information, but 77% had not attended any educational programmes on DV in the past year.

*Conclusions*: This study provides important information about current knowledge, attitudes, and beliefs of healthcare providers toward the diagnosis and management of DV. This information should prove useful to all who attempt to design clinical strategies and educational programmes to address this issue.

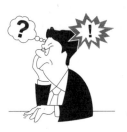

**Questions to think about**

1   What drawbacks can you foresee with the quantitative survey used in the study?
2   How far would your approach have addressed these concerns?
3   What advantage does the authors' approach offer?

We shall continue to develop the issue of methods in the following chapters.

## Evaluation and reflection

One of the key elements of any research study is the elimination of bias. In quantitative approaches, the attempt is made to eliminate bias. This worthy aim has a number of drawbacks. *It is probably impossible to eliminate bias in many real world situations.*

Researchers have a great ability for self-delusion in this area. The attempt to eliminate bias will often distort the situation or restrict its generalisability, particularly in the construction of RCTs.

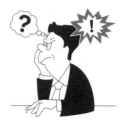

**Questions to think about**

1   Do you agree with these statements?
2   What perspective or bias do they contain?
3   Do you share this perspective, and does this affect your answer to question 1?

Within qualitative research, there is a less ambitious goal. The approach is generally:

• to identify and recognise bias within the researcher and research scenario
• to seek to minimise that bias, whilst not distorting the scenario itself
• evaluating the impact of that bias on the research scenario and researcher, and seeking to identify the impact on both the significance of the findings and their generalisability.

This may be regarded as either more realistic or defeatist according to your perspective or bias.

However, the recognition that bias exists is not an excuse for not minimising that bias. Rather, making it transparent should encourage researchers to re-double their efforts to minimise it. Pope, Ziebland and Mays (2000; cited in Chapter 11) consider the use of multiple researcher perspectives:

Some researchers have found that the use of more than one analyst can improve the consistency or reliability of analyses. However, the appropriateness of the concept of inter-rater reliability in qualitative research is contested. None the less there may be merit in involving more than one analyst in situations where researcher bias is especially likely to be perceived to be a problem, for example, where social scientists are investigating the work of clinicians. In a study of diagnosis in cardiology, Daly *et al.* developed a modified form of qualitative analysis involving external researchers and the cardiologists who had managed the patients. The researchers identified the main aspects of the consultations that seemed to be related to the use of echocardiography, and they developed criteria which other analysts could use to assess the raw data. The cardiologists then independently assessed each case using the raw data in order to produce an account of how and why a test was or was not ordered and with what consequences. The assessments of the cardiologists and researchers were compared statistically and the level of agreement was shown to be good.

Where there was disagreement between the original researchers' analysis and that of the cardiologist, a further researcher repeated the analysis and any remaining discrepancies were resolved by discussion between the researchers and the cardiologists. Although there was an element of circularity in part of this lengthy process (in that the formal criteria used by the cardiologists were derived from the initial researchers' analysis) and it involved the derivation of quantitative gradings and statistical analysis of inter-rater agreement that are unusual in a qualitative study, this process meant that clinical critics could not argue that the findings were simply based on the subjective judgements of an individual researcher.

Pope, Ziebland and Mays (2000)

However, it could be argued that such an approach is inconsistent with the qualitative approach, and a sop to the quantitative prejudices of some clinicians.

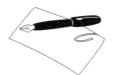

### Practical activities

1 Use your framework identified in Chapter 12 to evaluate the following study:

- Fletcher AE *et al.* (1999) Low uptake of eye services in rural India: a challenge for programs of blindness prevention. *Arch Opthalmol.* **117**: 1393–9.

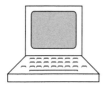

### On-line resource
You can access this paper via the Chapter 13 section of the website.

It is suggested that you produce your own evaluation framework based upon the Word version of the standard template downloadable from the website.

### Key points

By the end of this chapter, you should be able to:

1 Define a research question for a qualitative study.
2 Select appropriate methods for a qualitative study.
3 Evaluate bias and the researcher's own role in a qualitative study.

# 14

# Ethnography and grounded theory

## Introduction

The trouble with qualitative methods is that they have big words as names and this can be off putting. As an introduction, read Chapter 8 of:

- Pope C and Mays N (eds) (1999) *Qualitative Research in Health Care*. BMJ Books, London.

Then, for a more in-depth discussion of the process of grounded theory, read:

- Pandit NR (1996) The creation of theory: a recent application of the grounded theory method. *The Qualitative Report*. **2** (4).

- Dick B (2000) Grounded Theory: a thumbnail sketch. Available at http://www.scu.edu.au/schools/gcm/ar/arp/grounded.html

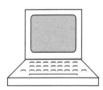

**On-line resource**
You can access all these papers via the Chapter 14 section of the website.

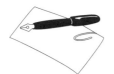

### Practical activities

1   Read the following model transcript that reflects (hypothetical-ish) interviews with clinicians in a hospital environment who were asked about the quality of information within their hospital trust.

---

'The biggest problem is the fact that we spend a lot of time putting information into computers and onto forms but when we want to access it it takes three days to get it, so we have to collect it again. It is very frustrating for the patients and the staff.'

'The IT staff aren't on a ward. They don't have a clue of the time pressure we're under.'

'There's no point in putting stuff on the computer. It just disappears.'

'Most of the information I want is held by social services.'

'The information that I gather from patients is confidential and I don't want to put into a big system where I don't know where it's going to end up.'

'I don't think I want to depend upon the data gathered by some of my colleagues.'

'The computers just gobble up information. They don't do anything for us.'

'The IT staff don't understand what we need as nurses.'

'Time spent filling in forms or at computers is time not spent on patients.'

'They've promised us a new computer system, but they've not asked us what we want, so I don't believe that it will do what I need.'

'They (the IT staff) live in a world of their own. I don't want access to NHS net, I want access to more nurses!'

'Computers are for the managers. They don't help doctors or patients.'

'They spent 6 billion pounds on IT, but I'm still filling in forms.'

'The idea of an integrated electronic patient record is great, but we're in the Dark Ages compared with that.'

'I use a word processor at home but we're still on paper forms on this ward.'

'A patient asked me the other day what happened to all the forms that we filled in. I didn't know.'

'I haven't got the time or the energy to learn how to use the computers. I'm too busy.'

'When I come on a night shift, it's very difficult to find out what's happened that day.'

'The IT staff are very helpful, but we don't see them very often.'

'I don't think the consultants are going to want to enter their own data at a keyboard, do you?'

2 Using the method outlined in *Grounded Theory: a thumbnail sketch* identify themes in the material.
3 Identify the core theme emerging from your transcript and the sub-themes related to that main theme.
4 What do you think your analysis is telling you about the respondents' views of the situation?

> **Warning!**
>
> This kind of analysis can't be fully appreciated from a small-scale exercise. If you would like to do some anger analysis of this type, then you will need to read the literature – there is a good bibliography in *Grounded Theory: a thumbnail sketch*. It's always a good idea to consult an experienced researcher who is familiar with these techniques.

5 Use your framework identified in Chapter 12 of this book to evaluate the following study:

• Martin DK, Thiel EC and Singer PA (1999) A new model of advance care planning: observations from people with HIV. *Arch Intern Med.* **159**: 86.

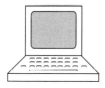

**On-line resource**
You can access this paper via the Chapter 14 section of the website.

# Action research on-line course

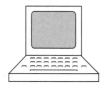

**On-line resource**
Hosted by the Southern Cross University in Northern New South Wales in Australia, there is an on-line action research course available at:

http://www.scu.edu.au/schools/gcm/ar/areol/
areolhome.html

This is, in fact, one part of a large website dedicated to action research, including journal articles, tutorials and conference presentations available at:

http://www.scu.edu.au/schools/gcm/ar/arhome.html

This site is available through the qualitative research resources section of the website, and is strongly recommended. Those thinking of doing their own research could well benefit from working through the course materials.

 **Key points**

By the end of this chapter, you should be able to:

1 Understand the principles of grounded theory and ethnographic analysis.
2 Identify themes within a transcript.
3 Be able to understand enough to undertake an analysis of a transcript under the supervision of an experienced researcher.

# 15

# Interview techniques

## Introduction

To start this chapter, read Chapter 8 of:

* Pope C and Mays N (eds) (1999) *Qualitative Research in Health Care*. BMJ Books, London.

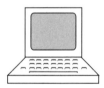

**On-line resource**
You can access this paper via the Chapter 15 section of the website.

Compare the advice with that given on grounded theory in Chapter 14 of this book.

---

Glaser recommends against recording or taking notes during an interview or other data collection session. Speaking for myself, I agree with his avoidance of tape recordings and word-by-word transcripts. I think you'll get more understanding from the extra interviews you could do in the time it would take you to listen to and transcribe a tape recording.

However, I think he is vulnerable on that point, and especially for thesis purposes. My suggestion is that you take key-word notes during the interviews and convert them to themes afterwards. I also suggest that you tape-record the interviews and check your notes against the tape recording. This won't be as time consuming (or alternatively, as costly) as full transcripts and in my experience it will do the job well.

If it's not for thesis purposes I think you can make your own choices. I neither take notes during interviews nor use a tape recorder. I find *rapport* develops more rapidly and effectively if I don't. However, I do have a memory system which allows me to memorise up to 20 distinct themes (more if it's necessary) and recall them in order.

Personal experience indicates that tape recording may prove a real barrier to frank responses, and may also generate a severe bout of data overload. There's no right answer. It's a matter of the optimum solution for your research problem.

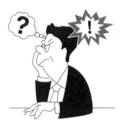

### Questions to think about

1　Would you find a tape recorder intimidating if you were being interviewed?
2　Under what circumstances?

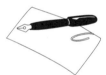

### Practical activities

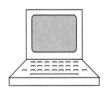

### On-line resource
There is an audio version of the transcript that can be downloaded from the Chapter 15 section of the website.

You will need to have sound on your PC to hear this, and a software application able to replay a .wav file.

1　In order to try transcribing an interview, listen to the audio version of the transcription from Chapter 14.
2　There are some minor transcription errors in the written version. Transcribe the audio version.
3　Compare the versions, and play 'spot the difference'!
4　Use your framework identified in Chapter 12 to evaluate the following study:

- Barrie R and Ward AM (1997) Questioning behaviour in general practice: a pragmatic study. *BMJ*. **315**: 1512–15.

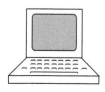

**On-line resource**
You can access this paper via the Chapter 15 section of the website.

**Key points**

By the end of this chapter, you should be able to:

1 Conduct an interview.
2 Transcribe an audio tape of an interview.
3 Appreciate the difficulties in carrying out interviews.

# 16

# Open-ended questionnaires for qualitative analysis

## Introduction

To consider the issue of questionnaires in a qualitative context first read:

- Snowdon C, Garcia J and Elbourne D (1998) Reactions of participants to the results of a randomised controlled trial: exploratory study. *BMJ*. **317**: 21–6.

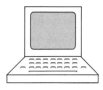

**On-line resource**
You can access this paper via the Chapter 16 section of the website.

## Questionnaires in a quantitative context

Questionnaires are a common research tool and may be used for quantitative or qualitative studies. The major difference between a questionnaire for quantitative or qualitative analysis is in the form of the questions. Questionnaires developed for quantitative analysis use closed questions.

For example:

Which of the following conditions do you believe poses the greatest risk to your health?

- breast cancer
- cervical cancer
- accidents
- coronary heart disease and strokes
- lung cancer.

This is a closed question. Its advantages are its ease of analysis and clarity of outcome. However, it is inflexible and makes assumptions about the respondents.

By comparison, a more open-ended question might be to ask the respondent the following:

---

Name the three conditions that you believe pose the greatest risk to your health?

1

2

3

Why?

---

This question has the advantage of allowing the respondent greater flexibility in response, and may provide a richer response. On the other hand it is more complex to analyse than the closed question. Many questionnaires in practice combine closed- and open-ended questions to get the best of both worlds. However, in such cases, the richness of the open-ended responses can be ignored because of the simplicity of analysing the closed questions.

## When is a questionnaire not a questionnaire?

In practice, questionnaires and interviews are not completely different animals. An open-ended question may be put to the respondent in a range of contexts, from a written questionnaire to an interview that may be conducted by phone, face-to-face or even by video conference.

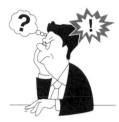

## Questions to think about

What are the advantages and disadvantages of a written questionnaire, telephone interview, video conference or face-to-face interview for asking open-ended questions?

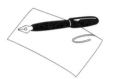

## Practical activities

1   Use your thoughts to fill in a table like the one below:

|  | *Advantages* | *Disadvantages* |
|---|---|---|
| Written questionnaire |  |  |
| Telephone interview |  |  |
| Video conference |  |  |
| Face-to-face interview |  |  |

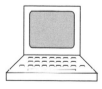

**On-line resource**
You can download a copy of this grid in Word or Acrobat format from the website.

2   The following recent studies, chosen for their diversity of topic, all used telephone interviews:

- Barrett PJ, Emmins PD, Clarke PD and Bradley DJ (1996) Comparison of adverse events associated with use of mefloquine and combination of chloroquine and proguanil as antimalarial prophylaxis: postal and telephone survey of travellers. *BMJ*. **313**: 525–8.
- Jeevaratnam DR and Menon DK (1996) Survey of intensive care of severely head injured patients in the United Kingdom. *BMJ*. **312**: 944–7.
- Keating NL, Cleary PD, Rossi AS *et al.* (1999) Use of hormone replacement therapy by postmenopausal women in the United States. *Ann Intern Med*. **130**: 545–53.
- Osmond DH, Catania J, Pollack L *et al.* (2000) Obtaining HIV test results with a home collection test kit in a community telephone sample. *J Acq Imm Def Synd*. **24**: 363–8.

Read the articles and answer the following questions for each study:

- Were any open-ended questions asked?
- What advantage would have been gained from the use of more open-ended questions?
- What disadvantages would there have been?
- What problems might have been experienced using a telephone survey for a more open-ended survey?
- Would a more open-ended survey from less respondents have produced a more useful result?

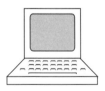

**On-line resource**
You can download a proforma for this exercise in Word or Acrobat format from the website.

3   Use your framework identified in Chapter 12 to evaluate the following study:

- Kumar S and Gantley M (1999) Tensions between policy makers and general practitioners in implementing new genetics: grounded theory interview study. *BMJ*. **319**: 1410–13.

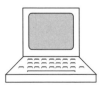

**On-line resource**
You can access this paper via the Chapter 16 section of the website.

**Key points**

By the end of this chapter, you should be able to:

1 Decide whether to use closed or open questions in a questionnaire.
2 Decide whether to use a written questionnaire or interview.
3 Evaluate the use of questionnaires in other studies.

# 17

# Focus groups

## Introduction

By way of introduction to this chapter, read Chapter 3 of:

- Pope C and Mays N (eds) (1999) *Qualitative Research in Health Care*. BMJ Books, London.

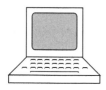

**On-line resource**
You can access this article via the Chapter 17 section of the website.

Focus groups are one of the most popular forms of qualitative research, and are regarded by many as 'trendy' and therefore judged in a negative manner. We shall explore the use of focus groups in this chapter by considering three studies that use focus groups in different ways.

## Study 1

Dolan P, Cookson R and Ferguson B (1999) Effect of discussion and deliberation on the public's views of priority setting in healthcare: focus group study. *BMJ.* **318**: 916–19.

Start by reading the article.

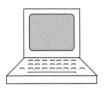

**On-line resource**
You can access this article via the Chapter 17 section of the website.

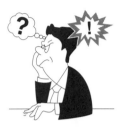

**Questions to think about**

1 How does this study use focus groups?
2 Do you think that the discussions were led, and if so, was it appropriate?
3 Do you agree with the study's findings?
4 Do you think that all topics would be as affected by discussion, and if so what are the implications for questionnaire surveys?

# Study 2

Hoddinott P and Pill R (1999) Qualitative study of decisions about infant feeding among women in the East End of London. *BMJ*. **318**: 30–4.

Start by reading the article.

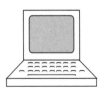

**On-line resource**
You can access this article via the Chapter 17 section of the website.

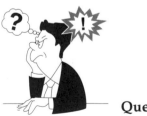

**Questions to think about**

1 How does this study use focus groups?
2 How does this differ from the last study?

3 What differences do you discern between responses in focus groups from those in individual interviews?
4 Do you think the focus groups added value to the study? Why?

# Study 3

Knudsen HC *et al.* (2000) Translation and cross-cultural adaptation of outcome measurements for schizophrenia. EPSILON Study 2. *Br J Psychr.* **177**: s8–s14.

Start by reading the article.

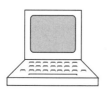

**On-line resource**
You can access this article via the Chapter 17 section of the website.

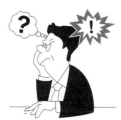

**Questions to think about**

1 How does this study use focus groups?
2 How do studies using clinicians differ from those studies based on patients?
3 How might this study have been done using other methods?
4 Do you think the focus groups achieved a better result? Why?

# Conclusions

These studies show that focus groups may be used in a wide variety of ways. They are often used in conjunction with other methods and the element of discussion and interaction can produce a different response. However, we should recognise that there are pitfalls and that a different response is not necessarily a 'better' response. The job of a facilitator is difficult. The interaction between contributors is the key to a successful focus group. If this interaction is what we seek to capture, then focus groups are a good way to gather data. However, if we are simply using them as a less resource-intensive replacement for one-to-one interviews, we are introducing another source of bias and uncertainty for no good reason.

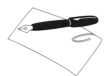

## Practical activities

1 Your senior partner or manager suggests that you should run a focus group to canvass patient opinions on the services that you provide.

   What information would you need to provide for the patients attending the session explaining the process and objectives, including any practical advice that you feel they may need?

   You may find it helpful to collect your thoughts as a written note to patients.
2 Use your framework identified in Chapter 12 to evaluate the three studies you have examined in this chapter.

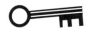 ## Key points

By the end of this chapter, you should be able to:

1 Evaluate a study based upon a focus group.
2 Understand the principles of running a focus group.
3 Evaluate the benefits of using a focus group in conjunction with other techniques.

# 18

# A combined approach

## Introduction

In *Qualitative Research in Health Care* (Pope C and Mays N (eds) (1999) BMJ Books, London) the issue of triangulation or multi-method approach is referred to:

---

Another feature of qualitative research (which some authors emphasise) is that it often employs several different methods or adopts a 'multi-method' approach. Watching people in their own territory thus entails observing, joining in (participant observation), talking with people (interviews, focus groups and informal chatting) and reading what they have written. In the healthcare context, a range of qualitative research methods has been employed to tackle important questions about social phenomena, ranging from complex human behaviours such as patients' compliance with treatment, and decision making by healthcare professionals, through to the organisation of the hospital clinic or of the NHS itself.

---

Increasingly, however, healthcare research is making use of qualitative and quantitative approaches within the same study.

## Combining different qualitative approaches

To consider how this may benefit a research study compare two qualitative studies. The first is based upon a single method, that of a semi-structured interview:

- Donovan JL and Blake DR (2000) Qualitative study of interpretation of reassurance among patients attending rheumatology clinics: 'just a touch of arthritis, doctor?' *BMJ*. **320**: 541–4.

Start by reading the article.

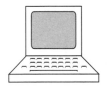

**On-line resource**
You can access this article via the Chapter 18 section of the website.

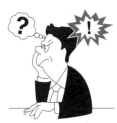

**Questions to think about**

1  How does the study use semi-structured interviews?
2  Could the study produce a richer perspective by combining the semi-structured interview with other methods?

Now consider the following study:

- Britten N *et al.* (2000) Misunderstandings in prescribing decisions in general practice: qualitative study. *BMJ*. **320**: 484–8.

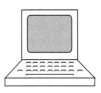

**On-line resource**
You can access this article via the Chapter 18 section of the website.

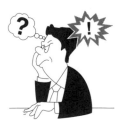

**Questions to think about**

1  How does the study use a variety of methods?
2  Does the combination of methods produce a better result? Why?

Triangulation is often cited as an essential part of qualitative research. However, it is very important that the purpose of triangulation is clear and the benefits realised.

# Mixing quantitative and qualitative approaches

Many healthcare studies benefit from combining qualitative and quantitative approaches. There are at least three types of combined approaches.

## *Using qualitative research to define hypotheses for a quantitative study*

Traditionally in medicine where the randomised controlled trial (RCT) is still seen as the 'gold standard' (see my presentation on RCTs for a discussion of this: we shall revisit this paper in the exercise at the end of the chapter), qualitative research is seen as a precursor to a quantitative study. The qualitative study seeks to refine the problem. This approach is often based upon prejudice that the findings of the qualitative study are not truly valid and therefore require validation by a 'proper' quantitative study. However, many of the problems amenable to qualitative research are simply not amenable to a RCT approach. Therefore, studies can distort situations in an attempt to produce a valid trial methodology.

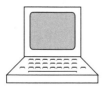

**On-line resource**
You can access my presentation on RCTs via the Chapter 18 section of the website.

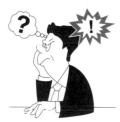

**Questions to think about**

1   Do you agree with the points made in the discussion on RCTs?
2   How do RCTs distort studies in order to make the study fit the model and not the other way around?

## *Using qualitative research to investigate the underlying reasons for findings from a quantitative study*

This is the reverse of the above. A quantitative study in a behavioural or policy context will often define what is going on. For example, the author was recently commissioned to investigate the recruitment of nurses from ethnic minorities. The result was a descriptive analysis of the situation. It revealed significant differences between recruitment of students from different ethnicities. However, it did not explain why recruitment from some ethnic minorities (e.g. Black African) was well above the proportion in the general population and in other cases (e.g. Bangladeshi) recruitment was almost non-existent.

Further quantitative analysis was able to reveal some further information. For example, it was possible to show that recruitment reflected applications, i.e. the inequalities were largely outside the actual recruitment process. However, the report concludes with the following section:

---

Therefore, further investigation is desirable to answer the following questions:

- Do students from ethnic minority backgrounds entering nursing wish to attend their nearest higher education institution (HEI)?
- What is the distribution of population concentrations of different ethnicities relative to the location of HEIs offering nursing courses?
- At what level of maturity can improved procedures be shown to lead to increased recruitment?
- What is the impact of overseas recruitment on the recruitment of UK nursing students from non-white ethnic minorities?
- What do actual and potential nursing students from these backgrounds perceive as the barriers to entry into the profession?
- What steps do actual and potential nursing students from these backgrounds perceive as effective in overcoming these barriers?
- What are factors that influence the differential recruitment between students of Asian and Afro-Caribbean ethnicity?
- Do lecturers regard equality of recruitment as a priority, or only as a requirement when overall recruitment falls?

Much of this would require qualitative research based around either semi-structured interviews or focus groups.

---

Crucially, if we are to understand the reasons why students from certain ethnicities are not applying for the nursing profession, this can only be achieved by a qualitative study. If the aim is to improve practice, then the reasons why are at least as significant as the actual situation. Therefore, in this case, we have used a quantitative study to establish the questions we wish to ask in a qualitative study.

The author has supervised a number of research degree projects of this type where the problem has been investigated quantitatively in the first stage of the investigation, up to MPhil level, and where a PhD phase has probed underlying reasons through interviews, case studies, focus groups or work shadowing.

## *Using qualitative and quantitative approaches in a single study*

In some studies, it will be possible to combine both approaches in a single study. Typical of this approach would be a questionnaire survey where closed questions that provide quantitative data are supplemented by open-ended questions that are designed to be analysed by textual analysis. In some cases, the open-ended questions may be better asked through an interview or focus group situation. This generally produces a much richer response than open-ended questions in a questionnaire survey.

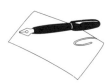

### Practical activities

Return to the paper in my presentation on RCTs cited earlier in the chapter. The first paper examined in the Introduction (Chapter 1) was:

*   Lattimer V *et al.* (1998) Safety and effectiveness of nurse telephone consultation in out of hours primary care: randomised controlled trial. *BMJ.* **317**: 1054–9.

Consider the reference that the authors make to a patient survey. If you were designing this study from scratch, how might you incorporate a mixed method approach to the problem?

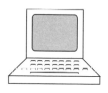

### On-line resource
You can access this article via the Introduction section of the website.

### Key points

By the end of this chapter, you should be able to:

1 Design a study incorporating qualitative and quantitative methods.
2 Design a study incorporating different qualitative methods.
3 Compare and contrast different qualitative approaches.

# Part Four
# Writing for research

# 19

# How to write a research proposal

## Introduction

There are many useful guides to writing research proposals on the Web. Before starting this chapter, you may like to refer to the following:

- Thackrey D (1997) University of Michigan's Division of Research and Development Administration.

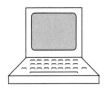
**On-line resource**
You can access this guide via the Chapter 19 section of the website.

## What makes a good proposal?

The first task is to find a suitable funding agency. In the UK primary care sector, this may well be the NHS. Whenever you seek funding, it is important to understand the funding agency's priorities, aims and objectives. For example, refer to the NHS R&D policy documents provided in the virtual library.

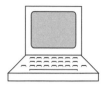

**On-line resource**
You can access this section of the virtual library via the Chapter 19 section of the website.

The framework that we have employed to evaluate published research can be adapted to help us plan a good proposal. A good proposal will show how it will deliver research, meeting all the criteria in our evaluation framework.

It is also worth noting reasons commonly cited for proposals being rejected:

*The application is outside the purview of the funding agency*
The applicant either failed to learn about the agency's restrictions or areas of interest or misunderstood them.

*The subject is not relevant to an issue of regional or national importance or lacks sufficient scientific significance*
Most funding agencies seek to fund projects which offer the prospect of replicable solutions to societal problems or that will make a significant contribution to knowledge in a particular field.

*The methodology appears to be flawed*
A proposal may address a problem of significance which is important to the funding agency, but it may be rejected because it approaches the problem in a way that the reviewers do not believe adequately tests its own assumptions or because it fails to ask the right questions.

*The applicant has not included measurable outcome indicators in the proposal*
Without some means of measuring the success of the project, funding agencies will not invest their resources.

*The funding agency is not the most appropriate source of funds for the proposed project*
If reviewers believe another Government program or private foundation is a more appropriate source of funding, they may decline a proposal regardless of its merits. In some cases, they will refer the grant seeker to the more appropriate source.

*The funding agency has already funded a similar project*
It is rare that a problem of regional or national and sometimes scientific significance is perceived in only one place at one time. If the funding agency has already funded someone else who has approached the same problem in the same general way, a turndown is likely.

*The funding agency's priorities and interests may have changed*
Because both governmental agencies and foundations are concerned with addressing changing societal problems or advancing technology, their priorities

and interests are constantly evolving. What was a priority a month ago may now have been replaced by an emerging issue.

*The proposed project does not allow for the highest and best use of the agency's funds*
Most funding agencies do not consider charitable effects of a proposed project as a major decision factor. Instead, they have goals of putting in place programmes which can be self-sustaining and can be replicated or which will have a major impact on a discipline.

*The applicant has failed to demonstrate fiscal accountability*
Funding agencies will make grants only to those organisations which have demonstrated ability to manage the funds. Failure to provide sufficient detail regarding fiscal systems and experience can result in a turndown.

*The applicant has used the 'shotgun' approach*
It is clear to reviewers when the applicant has not read or understood the agency's interests and application procedures and has instead forwarded a generic proposal to many funding sources at the same time. Lack of 'match' with the agency's priorities and criteria ensures a turndown.

A combination of these factors enables us to draw up a checklist which we can use to evaluate any proposal before submission:

---

### Checklist for a research proposal

*The academic perspective*

1  Is there a clearly formulated hypothesis? ☐

2  Is the proposed approach appropriate? ☐

3  Is the sampling strategy appropriate? ☐

4  What are the potential biases and have they been minimised? ☐

5  Does the proposal acknowledge the limits of the study? ☐

6  Methods (i) are they appropriate and described in enough detail? ☐

7  Methods (ii) what quality control measures were used? ☐

8  Is the planned programme likely to provide credible and significant results? ☐

9  Does the planned programme demonstrate the generalisability of the research? ☐

*The practitioner perspective*

1   Does the proposal demonstrate any obvious application that
could lead to an improvement in patient care?  ☐

2   Does the proposed research have relevance to everyday
patient care?  ☐

*The management perspective*

1   Does the proposal show how it may generate evidence that
could be disseminated?  ☐

2   Does the proposal suggest how any resulting evidence could
be disseminated?  ☐

3   Would the application of the proposed research have a
positive or negative economic impact?  ☐

*The strategic perspective*

1   Does the proposed research explain the underlying reasons for
events?  ☐

2   Will the research assist in the delivery of national NHS strategies?  ☐

*The funder's perspective*

1   Is the application outside the purview of the funding agency?  ☐

2   Is the subject relevant to an issue of regional or national
importance or does it lack sufficient scientific significance?  ☐

3   Has the applicant included measurable outcome indicators
in the proposal?  ☐

4   Is the funding agency the most appropriate source of
funds for the proposed project?  ☐

5   Has the funding agency already funded a similar project?  ☐

6   Have the funding agency's priorities and interests changed?  ☐

7   Does the proposed project allow for the highest and best use
of the agency's funds?  ☐

8   Has the applicant demonstrated fiscal accountability?  ☐

9   Has the applicant demonstrated a match to the funder's aims
and objectives?  ☐

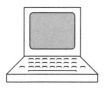

**On-line resource**
You can download an Acrobat or Word version of this checklist from the Chapter 19 section of the website.

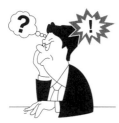

**Questions to think about**

1  Which research areas that you are interested in are likely to be priority areas for a potential funder?
2  Why?

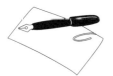

**Practical activities**

Read the sample proposal available from the website.

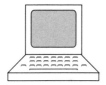

**On-line resource**
You can download a copy of the sample proposal from the Chapter 19 section of the website.

• Evaluate the proposal in terms of the checklist.
• Would you fund the work?

 **Key points**

By the end of this chapter, you should be able to:

1  Critically evaluate a research proposal.
2  Design a research proposal.

# 20

# Writing a research report

## Introduction

By now, you should have a pretty good idea of what is required for a good research article. In this chapter we shall work through a series of activities to reinforce your knowledge. For detailed information about the requirements of a specific journal refer to the advice to contributors usually found on the journal website.

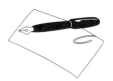

**Practical activities**

Use the World Wide Web to compare the instructions to authors given by the *BMJ* with those for *JAMA* and another journal of your choice accessed on-line.

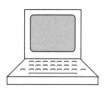

**On-line resource**
The Chapter 20 section of the website includes links to key journals for primary care, including *JRCGP*, *BMJ*, *JAMA*, *NEJM*.

Record your answers in a table such as the one overleaf:

| General instructions | Journal specific instructions | | |
|---|---|---|---|
| | *BMJ* | *JAMA* | |
| Abstract style | | | |
| Format | | | |
| Word length | | | |
| Referencing system | | | |
| Other | | | |

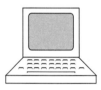

**On-line resource**
The Chapter 20 section of the website includes proformas of this table in Acrobat and Word format.

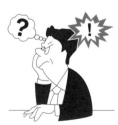

**Questions to think about**

Re-visit the paper we evaluated in the Introduction. Using the knowledge that you have gained reading the book, re-evaluate the paper.

1 Have your conclusions changed in either nature or strength?
2 Has your understanding been fundamentally changed or merely amplified and clarified in key areas?
3 Do you feel more confident in your evaluation of the paper?

**Key points**

By the end of this chapter, you should be able to:

1   Critically evaluate a research paper.
2   Write up a piece of research.
3   Evaluate your own learning whilst reading this book.

# 21

# Conclusions:
# evidence from research

## Introduction

The workbook *Providing Information for Health* has a lot of detailed information about evidence-based healthcare. In this chapter we shall only consider the link between research and evidence. In particular, we shall consider the commonly used definition of 'evidence'. First, read David Sackett's editorial in the *BMJ* on evidence-based medicine:

- Sackett DL, Rosenberg WMC, Muir Gray JA *et al.* (1996) Evidence based medicine: what it is and what it isn't. *BMJ.* **312**: 71–2.

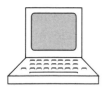

**On-line resource**
You can access this article from the Chapter 21 section of the website.

## What is evidence-based healthcare?

Evidence-based medicine, or evidence-based healthcare as it has become known, is based on the principle that doctors should act in accordance with the best evidence available. It sounds deceptively simple and a proposition that few could argue with. Further, the whole rationale for doing research within the NHS has become the desire to provide new evidence in order to improve healthcare practice and, hopefully, the health of patients.

Unfortunately, there are a number of problems:

- the evidence is not always available
- it may not be clear how strong the evidence is
- the best evidence may not apply to the patient concerned because of age, sex or confounding factors
- evidence gathering usually involves meta-analysis, which has its own problems
- evidence may be seen as an unwelcome imposition by managers or external agencies, leading to resistance especially where issues of health economics are involved.

Some practitioners are seeking to recognise the ambiguities inherent in this simple concept. Consider the following article by Dr Nicholas Hicks in *Bandolier*:

---

David Sackett's definition of 'evidence-based medicine' (EBM) is now well known and widely accepted. But the phrase 'evidence-based healthcare' (EBHC) is rarely defined. Much of my work involves explaining and trying to apply the principles of EBM and EBHC, often to people who have been puzzled and even irritated by what they had thought EBM and EBHC implied about their current and past practice. I have evolved my explanation of EBHC into a definition:

> 'Evidence-based healthcare takes place when decisions that affect the care of patients are taken with due weight accorded to all valid, relevant information.'

Several things follow from this definition:

1 'Decisions that affect the care of patients' are taken by managers and health policy makers as well as by clinicians. EBHC is therefore just as relevant to managers and policy makers as it is to clinicians.
2 'Due weight' implicitly acknowledges that there are many factors that contribute to decisions about the care of patients. There are many factors other than the results of randomised controlled trials (RCTs) that may weigh heavily in both clinical and policy decisions (for instance, patient preferences and resources). This definition requires that valid, relevant evidence should be considered alongside other relevant factors in the decision-making process. It does not assume that any one sort of evidence should necessarily be the determining factor in a decision.
3 'All' is aspirational – but it implies that there should be an active search for valid, relevant information.
4 'Valid, relevant' implies that before information is used in a decision, an

assessment should be made of the accuracy of the information and the applicability of the evidence to the decision in question; that is, information should be appraised.

5 'Information' is deliberately left unspecified; there are many types of information that may be valid and relevant in particular circumstances. I have no wish to exclude any particular type of information as long as an appraisal is made of its validity and relevance and the information is given 'due weight' – neither more nor less.

Other things follow from this definition, not least that the concept of EBHC is not new – it's what most people I know have been trying to practise all their working lives. But there are new reasons and new opportunities to help us improve the care that patients receive, including:

- more and better information, e.g. from the increasing number of well-conducted RCTs and systematic reviews
- the better organisation of information and new insights that derive from the evolving science of systematic review
- rapid advances in information technology
- an improving (though still inadequate) understanding of the (social and organisational) processes by which research findings are translated into practice.

I have been using this definition for a year or so now. People seem to find it useful and non-threatening.

---

This definition recognises some of the inherent ambiguities in evidence-based practice. However, more traditional evidence-based approaches define hierarchies of evidence, such as:

| Level | Evidence type |
|---|---|
| I | Strong evidence from at least one published systematic review of multiple well-designed RCTs |
| II | Strong evidence from at least one published properly designed RCT of appropriate size and in an appropriate clinical setting |
| III | Evidence from published well-designed trials without randomisation, single group pre-post cohort, time series or matched case-controlled studies |
| IV | Evidence from well-designed non-experimental studies from more than one centre or research group |
| V | Opinions of respected authorities, based on clinical evidence, descriptive studies or reports of expert consensus committees |

In primary care, for the majority of patients, a relatively small number of conditions have evidence above level IV. Even in secondary care, studies are emerging that show many guidelines and benchmarks are at best based upon evidence at level III, and often IV.

A simple illustration of the problem are drug trials that for reasons of trial design usually specifically exclude pregnant women, children and patients aged over 65 years. These are the very groups that are presenting most often in general practice.

The evidential hierarchy fails to acknowledge qualitative research except as descriptive studies at the lowest level, since it is not in the traditional sense of the word, 'generalisable'.

These problems have led to some frustration amongst clinicians. See, for example:

- Isaacs D and Fitzgerald D (1999) Seven alternatives to evidence-based medicine. *BMJ.* **319**: 1618.

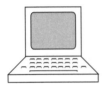

### On-line resource
You can access this article from the Chapter 21 section of the website.

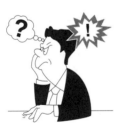

### Questions to think about

1   Compare the definition of EBHC by Dr Hicks with the evidential hierarchy. Is there a conflict here?
2   If the whole rationale for doing research within the NHS is to provide new evidence in order to improve healthcare practice and, hopefully, the health of patients, what value is there in qualitative research, and should the NHS be funding it?

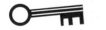 ### Key points

By the end of this chapter, you should be able to:

1   Define and comment on the validity of the evidential hierarchy.
2   Distinguish between evidence-based healthcare and evidence-based medicine.
3   Read a research paper and assess its evidential value.

# Index